A Family Disease

A Family Disease

A Memoir of Multigenerational Ataxia

DANA LORENE CREIGHTON

Foreword by
John F. Evans, MAT, MA, Ed.D.

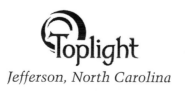

Jefferson, North Carolina

LIBRARY OF CONGRESS CATALOGUING-IN-PUBLICATION DATA

Names: Creighton, Dana Lorene, 1973– author.
Title: A family disease : a memoir of multigenerational ataxia / Dana
Lorene Creighton ; foreword by John F. Evans, MAT, MA, Ed.D.
Description: Jefferson, North Carolina : Toplight, 2021 | Includes
bibliographical references and index.
Identifiers: LCCN 2020054446 | ISBN 9781476683188 (paperback : acid free paper) ∞
ISBN 9781476641959 (ebook)
Subjects: LCSH: Creighton, Dana Lorene, 1973—Health. |
Ataxia—Patients—United States—Biography. | Ataxia—Genetic aspects. |
Genetic disorders.
Classification: LCC RC376.5 .C74 2021 | DDC 616.8/3—dc23
LC record available at https://lccn.loc.gov/2020054446

BRITISH LIBRARY CATALOGUING DATA ARE AVAILABLE

ISBN (print) 978-1-4766-8318-8
ISBN (ebook) 978-1-4766-4195-9

Front cover artwork *In Her City* © 2021 by Sarah Goodyear

Printed in the United States of America

Toplight is an imprint of McFarland & Company, Inc., Publishers

*Box 611, Jefferson, North Carolina 28640
www.toplightbooks.com*

Acknowledgments

The National Ataxia Foundation (NAF) provided a wealth of information that I was thankful to have access to. Through it (ataxia. org), I sought and found connections to others who had a shared passion for living with hope. Making numerous connections over the past 10 years through it and hearing others' stories laid a foundation for me being compelled to share my family's story. I have made meaningful connections with numerous people in the Ataxia community. Hearing how others told their own narratives allowed me to broaden the range of experiences that unites us all. Having Ataxia and a family story affected by it only made relating to others in all kinds of situations and conditions easier.

Reading and digesting dozens of personal stories helped me reconstruct my own rocky journey. The more I wrote, the more clearly it became apparent that we are all more similar than different. Fortunately, even though I did not even know what exactly I was searching for, John Evans came along. He had the wisdom and insight to see what I needed to do and helped guide me toward it. His support led me to finding my way on this path. There are dozens of positive connections I made through my basketball career. From fourth grade through college, there were teammates, coaches, opponents, idols, rivals and fans who helped contour my experiences. There may be as many influential people who show up as characters in my story as those who do not. I am eternally grateful this is the case. I don't think my story could have happened any other way. Whether a character is listed in my story or absent from it, I acknowledge their contribution to my life.

Acknowledgments

I am grateful for the love of my brothers and parents who helped me learn to shape love into all of my experiences. I want to thank my dad's family who offered constant support and a positive presence to me throughout my life. Thank you seems too simple a phrase to say to my mom's family who have countless heart-wrenching stories about loved ones that live on in their minds. Thank you for sharing some of them with me and introducing me to their spirits. I'm so grateful we found each other again.

Table of Contents

Table of Contents

Foreword

by John F. Evans

A Family Disease is a memoir about hope, faith, the power of connection and writing to heal. It is about learning the language your mother speaks to you after she is gone from your life. You understand her better now because you already know her language, and you realize you always knew it. You know it by heart; it's in your blood.

This work actually began about four years ago as a result of a chance meeting between a man and a woman who would resume roles they had played years before as coach and athlete. As I remember it now, it was a warm spring day in 2016 at the Forest Hills tennis courts in Durham, North Carolina, where my son was taking tennis lessons with several other kids his age. Parents were gathered along the fence or sitting in their cars. As I looked for my friend, whose boy was also at lessons, I noticed a tall, athletic-looking woman with short blonde hair talking with a young African American girl about 10, my son's age, holding a tennis racket. I had seen the girl and her father before at the tennis lessons but had not met her mother. As the woman turned from the girl, I could see a big smile on her face, and I wondered to myself why this woman looked familiar to me. (She reminded me of a girl who had played center for me when I coached high school basketball. I guessed she played at 6'1", 170, a collegiate forward. As it turns out, I wasn't far off.) When the girls and boys entered the tennis courts, the parents gathered in the spectator area, and I had to satisfy my curiosity about this familiar-looking person. As I walked over to where she was standing, I said, "I think I know you from somewhere but I can't remember." Without hesitation, she laughed and said, "I'm Dana Creighton. I was in your Expressive Writing for Resilience study at Duke Integrative Medicine from January to March this year."

I told Dana that I would love to hear about her experience in the study because as I was the co-investigator and facilitator, protocol did not provide me an opportunity to talk with anyone who participated. Dana said she was "surprised that her experience was such a good one, because I don't consider myself a writer." She went on to say she found the writing to be very beneficial still after a couple of months. We continued to talk through the tennis lesson about her experience in the study and how it reminded her of research about health coaches she had coordinated. As we talked more about research, writing, and health coaching, Dana said she was thinking she might like to work with a health coach, so I stepped into the breach and admitted I was a health coach and I would love to work with her. We saw what our calendars allowed.

The next week, Dana and I met and developed a plan for her to set some goals and create space for new things she wanted in her life. As we developed Dana's plan, executed it, and set new goals and plans, it became obvious to me that there were more ways that Dana could employ writing to heal strategies and that her story was an incredible one of love, courage and strength.

As I learned more about Dana's life, a pattern emerged. It was a pattern of family tragedy followed by silence and silent questions answered by more silence. Dana learned the language of silence by immersion. Something I learned as I worked with her is that Dana is also a researcher at heart and a good one.

Tirelessly, Dana sought answers to family secrets, and there she learned her mother's language, her mother's tongue. Dana traveled through time and space to tell a story about her family tragedy that no one had ever put together. She gathered photographs, letters, notes, books and songs. She interviewed countless people, including her cousins, aunts, brothers, and her father. From a researcher's perspective I might write: "This book is an extension of an expressive writing prompt four years ago when I met with 39 participants in a research project at Duke Integrative Medicine. Dana was a member of that group of subjects in the study. This is her story."

But the book you are holding in your hands is more than that. Dana and I have met more than 120 times in the last three years, each time meeting for at least an hour. I have learned from Dana. She makes her coach look good in these pages. In the process of talking and writing, we have laughed and cried and pondered the great questions of what it means to be human, to be a man, to be a woman, to live, to love, to lose, to go, to stay, to forgive, to let go, to have a friend, to be a friend, to have a family, to be a family, to suffer and to thrive. In the way we all have of sharing these human conditions, this is your story too because as you spend time reading it, you will learn the language with which to face challenges with hope, courage, compassion, nonjudgment, faith, loving kindness, and the power of connection.

John F. Evans, MAT, MA, Ed.D., is an expressive writing clinician, expressive writing researcher, and national board-certified health and wellness coach, who teaches groups, individuals and healthcare professionals how to use writing for better physical, emotional and spiritual health. An author of five books, he has taught journaling and writing for self-development for more than 35 years.

Preface

This book bridges the enormous gap between the patient experience of illness and the sometimes impersonal aims of the clinician. After writing my story, it is obvious that the healthcare system had failed my mom and me in different ways. Unlike my mother, I had the right tools to piece together both meaning and purpose for my life. In this memoir I use bodies of research about neuroplasticity and inherited family trauma to demonstrate how our minds guide our intentions.

Medical records, personal correspondence and verbal accounts of my mother's family are used to uncover their story and ultimately mine. Comparing my own life experience with my mother's allows me to not only make sense of her life but also her death. The effect of a disease on family goes beyond the illness itself and into the very fabric of what family means. Being a forty-something mom with an adolescent daughter is a parallel that I share with my mom. How we each tell our stories influences what, when, and how we communicate illness to our daughters.

This intimate story is for anyone who has sought a medical opinion and received a tone-deaf reply. It is for women or men who have had to silently suffer through ambiguous loss—after losing a pregnancy or having an abortion. It is for the women who have been left by their partner after identifying their own illness or that of their child. It is for mental health professionals who have clients who have undergone a trauma but may not be capable of expressing their pain or of making sense of what has happened to them.

Sometimes we do not have the words to describe our trauma.

Others' inability to visibly grasp what we see does not keep it from infiltrating our experience of life. It is for practitioners who use and teach narrative medicine. Narratives help both patients and doctors understand the human dimension of disease beyond diagnosis and therapy, such as pain, suffering, family dynamics, and the meaning of illness. This story is also for those who need to deal with their own mortality or that of a loved one. Eventually you and everyone you love will die. Every life on this earth ends in death. But it does not have to be the last sentence in our story.

I have an MS in exercise physiology and have contributed to various scientific journals. I worked in medical research and community health at UNC–Chapel Hill and Duke University for nearly 20 years. I created a niche which involved taking apart the steps in a complex process to determine how to best implement an intervention. My mom's story was brought to life using these same tools to make sense of how our drastically different experiences and outcomes with the same disease became our reality. Since leaving the workforce in 2017, I volunteer with the National Ataxia Foundation (ataxia.org).

Introduction

An inherited neurologic disease was hovering over my family like a storm for more than 100 years. Like a tornado, it destroyed, injured, and maimed everyone in its path. This is a story of how my life was impacted by this condition—on my terms and from my perspective. I was entrenched in my own interpretation of witnessing my mom's struggle with the realities of this condition. I learned in researching her family that each of my mom's four siblings shared this affliction, all inheriting it from their father. Information I gathered from my mom's life helped me simulate her story which had escaped me for the majority of mine. I knew there was something unusual surrounding the lives and deaths of those on my mom's side. Something scary and secret.

I spent my childhood and adolescence witnessing what my mom's disease and confirmed diagnosis did to her emotionally. For the first five years or so I was simply watching my mom go about her life in the best way she could. She had symptoms, but I didn't really notice. I also didn't know at that time how her diagnosis devastated and challenged her will to live her life as she had so far. Right around this time I had a big diversion that helped shape my brain. I completely submerged my mind and body into the game of basketball for the next 15 years.

I was just about to begin my second year playing college ball when my mom committed suicide. After I had completed my final basketball season, I lost my sense of purpose. Until then, basketball was eating up nearly all my physical and mental energy, and I succumbed to my first bout of deep depression. At a time when I felt very lost and disconnected, I started a deep and nurturing relationship. I had found the sister and mother figure that I had secretly always wished for, one who provided her total support and unconditional love.

After I finished my degrees, I rarely read for pleasure. But when I did, I picked nonfiction. I started reading more and more and this trend continued for 20 years. I read dozens of memoirs that helped me find a vocabulary and my voice. After moving to North Carolina and for the next 19 years, I continued building deep connections within my close circle of friends. My girlfriends and all our children are a simulation of one larger family unit. Very early in my career, I had the privilege of working for a superb nurse, researcher, and person. I learned valuable lessons while working for her and the entire team.

In both research and nursing, if it didn't get documented, it didn't happen. I kept a paper trail of everything I could, just like my mom did, which was the only way to try and piece together what happened throughout her life then taking that information and truly trying to understand what was happening from her perspective. A few months after that dreadful September 11, I met my future husband in Durham. We eventually married with the intention of starting family. Weeks after we married in 2006, I got my own diagnosis. The same diagnosis that led to so much turmoil for my mom and her family. After a series of serious challenges to begin our own family, we adopted our daughter in 2008.

I attended church semi-regularly, albeit inconsistently, after our daughter was born. I also began really connecting with certain music, which inconspicuously and unconsciously allowed me to practice my own form of spirituality, helping me garner some hope. After my divorce I thought that it was so refreshing to be around people who knew the real me—my friends and all our kids. They didn't judge me, and they embraced all of me, all the time. I had no reason to hide anything from them and I didn't try to. I opened up to everyone I was close with, all that I had been through, and I wasn't afraid of being myself or holding anything back.

———————

During this same time, I was slowly progressing and hyperaware of each weakness I had, especially at work. As I started trying to prepare for what I might be asked to do, I wanted to be up front about my ability or inability to do it. I knew it was becoming increasingly uncomfortable to complete my work-related tasks. I was open and frank with my supervisor that I wasn't comfortable drawing blood anymore. It had been four years since I had been asked to do this and I had agreed to do it at that time. Meanwhile, I maintained strong family ties on my dad's side. Then our family reconnected with my cousins on my mom's side about the same time I started writing about my life. I had become accustomed to shrouding my pain in silence. I found out that telling my story could also be healing. My story reframed has given me a sense of calm and clarity about my past and my future.

I know that this isn't the entire story. It is my story in terms that are relevant and important to me. I will have to admit that writing it sometimes seemed more like a piece of fiction. After I had nearly finished, I saw something I never would have anticipated upon starting. My story is part adventure, part mystery, and at the backbone of my own narrative is a love story. The love I have received my entire life from my family provided a foundation—a foundation that allowed the love and gratitude I have to encompass each person that has touched my life in a profound way.

After knowing all that happened, I was the exact same person I had always been, but with the added wisdom that a career in research had given me and the ability to extrapolate a lifetime of seemingly separate and non-related events into a story of who, what, why and how. When the possibility of applying for disability came up, it was an option that did not come easily for me. By letting go of my career that I had been clinging to I was fortunate enough to be able to direct all my time and energy into trying to make some sense of the experiences of my life and my mother's. No longer working, I was able to dive headfirst into what I had always been compelled to do—discover what I could do to help others feel less alone.

CHAPTER I

What Comes Next

The only thing that makes life possible is permanent, intolerable uncertainty: not knowing what comes next.—*Ursula K. Le Guin,* The Left Hand of Darkness

THE FAMILY SECRET

Brian was the first sibling to accidentally find out that our family would be called up to the plate next. He was simply going to the bathroom late one evening, and as he passed my parents' bedroom, he overheard their strained and urgent back and forth commentary about something obviously painful and awful based on their tone. Mom was clearly distraught as she sobbed, "What are we going to do?" My dad, who was typically even tempered and overly rational, replied that they would just figure it out as they went. That was Brian's secret to carry, but not for long.

In December 1982, my dad explained to all four of us kids about our mom's confirmation of having the family disease. My dad called a family meeting and explained to all of us that Mom was finally diagnosed with the family disease. In his explanation, he included that it was dominantly inherited and was tailored for my two oldest brothers who were approaching adulthood. Our first cousin Mike saw symptoms as early as 12, and cousins Susie and Betsy were symptomatic in their early teens. Todd and Brian had already escaped their teen years unscathed. Scott was 11 and I was only 9. I'm certain that my mom played out the worst-case scenario in her mind which was that surely Scott or Dana would fall victim first.

I remember vividly that my first cousin Mike died while I was in the fifth grade and I knew he died at age 31 from the family disease in 1984. I remember standing in line in my elementary school cafeteria to get my lunch while considering that it was such a tragedy, but as I had no personal connection to anyone in Mike's immediate family, I went on with my day as usual. Mike's younger sister Vickie is now 60. I would call her randomly and frequently while I was trying to figure out Mom's story. I called her specifically so she could tell me about her brother Mike—a local cousin that I had never even met. Vickie told me in that phone conversation that Mike was

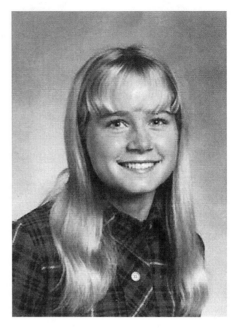

Susie Poynter, eighth grade, Kokomo, Indiana 1969.

a kind-hearted and wonderful older brother. Vickie was in his room at the nursing home every day for the last month of Mike's life. She spent her 26th birthday in the funeral home.

I have called my brother Brian numerous times over the last few years to help me piece together my mom's story. "What can you tell me from your recollection of the time period leading up to Mom's diagnosis?" He would have been 16 in 1981 and recalls Mom's denial while she was peeling potatoes in the kitchen. Mom stopped what she was doing, turned to him, paused and said, "You may have noticed that I am awkward sometimes when I move, but really I'm just clumsy." Brian had observed some of his cousins display symptoms of the disease. He had also noticed the same unco-ordinated, clunky movements that my mom was referring to. With little belief that he felt otherwise, he replied "OK" and carried

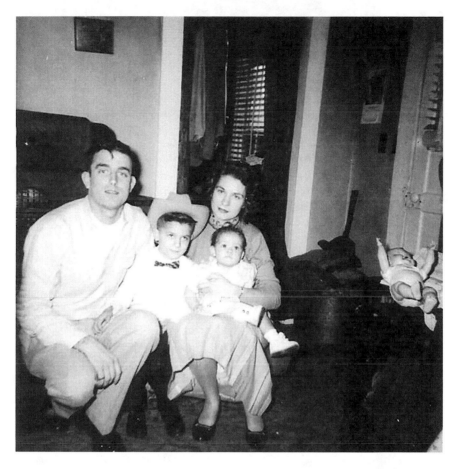

The Poynters, Bill and Anita, with children Mike and Vickie, at Christmas in Kokomo, Indiana, 1958.

on as if she had told him that it looked like it was going to rain today.

Still seeking more about the family secret, I called Cathy Creighton in the fall of 2017. She was my cousin and Mom's niece who was closer in age to Mom. Cathy told me that she remembers going out to eat when Mom shared her recent diagnosis, in early 1983. She said Mom fell down outside after leaving the restaurant. I could imagine the overwhelming feelings spewing out of control inside her, making the simple task of walking difficult as her energy was tied up in her emotions, not concentrating on coordinating each step. Months before I talked to Cathy, I had read *The Brain That Changes Itself* by Norman Doidge. After talking to her I was compelled to read it again, when the following text nearly jumped off the page.

> The mental "tracks" that get laid down can lead to habits, good or bad. If we develop poor posture, it becomes hard to correct. If we develop good habits, they too become solidified. Is it possible, once "tracks" or neural pathways have been laid down, to get out of those paths and onto different ones? Yes, according to Pascual-Leone, but it is difficult because, once we have created these tracks, they become "really speedy" and very efficient at guiding the sled down the hill. To take a different path becomes increasingly difficult. A roadblock of some kind is necessary to help us change direction [209].

Penny was also a close friend of my mom's and a definite roadblock in Mom's track that she was speeding down. I reached out to Penny before I started writing this book and many times since. She filled me in on much of the history of her relationship with my mom, as their friendship began years before I was born. In the mid–1960s,

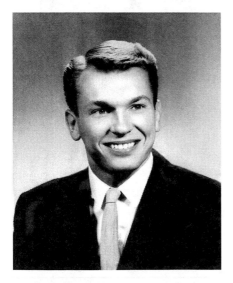

Robert Creighton, Indiana Central, Indianapolis, 1962.

Penny and Mom would drop off Todd and Brian with the babysitter, then commute together to Manchester College. Mom already had a business degree from Indiana Central in Indianapolis, where she met my dad. She decided to get another one, this time in home economics.

Almost 20 years later, Penny would reassure her that she was there for her then and always would be. My mom would not take her word for it, as she knew that close friends of her siblings would eventually wander further away as the disease progressed.

Mom stopped attending church, family get-togethers, and my sporting events. She eventually chose to be in the driver's seat and cut ties with each and every friend she had built connections with. My mom's decision to sever her personal connections affected all of us. Creating isolation from family and friends' comfort and support over the next 10 years would not just affect my mom. Just as much as my mom felt she was protecting herself from more pain, she was exposing the rest of our family to more. Over time my mom was training her neural pathways to do less and less physically and emotionally. We didn't talk about her ongoing absences or acknowledge them. We had all bought into keeping her secret.

MINDFULNESS

I was 10 years into living with my own diagnosis in 2016. My family disease had also been genotyped and named Spinocerebellar Ataxia Type 2 (SCA2). There have been more than 50 types of Ataxia identified since the early 1990s. Each steadily steals more and more of the control over most every aspect of life in its own way. The cerebellum is the part of the brain that controls important body functions. Ataxia causes gradual degeneration of this control center. Fine motor skills, coordination and balance will get progressively worse, until eventually swallowing and breathing will become impossible. Age of onset can differ greatly within the same type and rate of progression varies too.

Since I had been working at Duke University since 2009, I had utilized massage, yoga and craniosacral therapy at Duke Integrative Medicine (DIM). Craniosacral therapy is a light touch approach that releases tension deep in the body to relieve pain and dysfunction and improve whole body health. I had been working at Duke for different departments as a research coordinator, and I had coordinated a pilot study on health coaching and risk of heart disease at the Duke IM building which was freestanding and separate from the busy medical center. I enjoyed the ample, free parking and the serene and earthy vibe inside.

I was involved in all the phases of the study, but I spent most of my time training the health coaches on the study protocol. We mostly talked about logistics of the patient and coach relationship, but in doing so, I gained insight as to what they did and how they did it. I also recruited and scheduled baseline and follow-up visits for all the participants throughout the study. I ended up getting direct feedback about their reactions to the coaching, which was largely positive.

For months, I attended meetings with Dr. Ruth Wolever, the principal investigator (PI) of the study, who led our weekly team meetings. This was a typical scenario for almost every research project I was assigned to for the last 15 years, but Ruth was not a typical PI. She believed in getting things done efficiently and following proper protocol, but she said things exactly how they were and didn't candy coat anything. She has an incredible spirit and is funny as hell. She is also a mother of a severely handicapped daughter. I admired Ruth for her leadership and professional accomplishments but even more so for her ability to speak freely about her family's circumstances along with the dedication and love she showed for her daughter.

I worked with another coordinator who was also one of the study's health coaches. Since I was new to how health coaching worked, I directed most of my questions to her. This experience opened my mind to even more possibilities as health coaching was relatively new. I was completely on board with the benefits it could produce. But I was certain I would never need one. Five years after learning what it was, I decided I not only needed but wanted one. I thought I was living a pretty healthy lifestyle exercise- and nutrition-wise. I didn't have a specific area that I felt needed attention, but my health coach John assured me we would find what we were looking for. We started small and took baby steps. When we met for the first time and he suggested I start with "mindfulness" I immediately bought in, knowing mine had a lot of room for improvement. We agreed to develop a program of yoga as a means to practice it. This road seemed incredibly safe. A health coach in Atlanta gives this example of how health coaching was designed to work.

> We help people take big goals and break them down into accessible,
> bite-size pieces—not by telling clients what to do but by helping clients
> figure out what will work for them. Health coaching gets to the heart
> of what providing good health care is about: acceptance, partnership,
> compassion, and helping patients feel respected and understood [*New
> York Times*, Jan. 7, 2020].

John and I utilized "health coaching" in a very loose way. By the book, health coaching is highly structured, but we were all over the map and almost never had a set agenda. From the moment I would walk into his office, one of us would just spontaneously erupt into a new topic. Wanting to think through my mom's story from her perspective was looming over me like a shadow. It had been for so long that it felt like a part of me. I was unable to see it separate from myself until eventually verbalizing it with John.

Throughout my life, my mom's story remained a mystery to me. I couldn't even make a story up that might help me make sense of hers. I was only partially aware of what my mom had endured within her own family through 2016. It became a personal mission to find out how it happened that my mom, who had proven to be resilient for more than half of her life, made the choice to end her suffering once and for all. This subject would take over my discussions with John. Once this ball started rolling downhill, I couldn't have stopped it if I tried.

I am by nature quiet and introverted and typically a great listener, not a talker. However, I could not stop talking with John as there were so many aspects of my own condition that I had questions about and needed to explore the possibilities. He was there to listen to me and learn what was important to me. John and I would pose different questions about what happened in myself and what had happened to my mom physically and emotionally. We started out with focusing on being more mindful and ended up somewhere else.

It wasn't until I started talking about my and Mom's life that I even came up with a probable story. I discovered several parallels in our lives. I lived my life building and maintaining strong family connections, and Mom lived hers with disintegrating ones. This was due in part to death, but also to Mom's perception that her family did not exhibit the standards that she valued. If that wasn't enough to keep them at arm's length, the family disease certainly was. By talking through with my health coach the mechanisms that had been helpful to me, I realized over time that they were the very things that led my mom down the road of despair.

Eventually John and I explored discoveries in neuroplasticity through articles and books. When we first discussed *The Brain That Changes Itself* by Norman Doidge, I chose to watch the documentary which left me exhilarated and hungry to delve deeper into the implications of neuroplasticity. Here is an excerpt explaining neuroplasticity and its history.

> *Neuro* is for "neuron," the nerve cells in our brains and nervous systems. *Plastic* is for "changeable, malleable, modifiable." At first many of the scientists didn't dare use the word "neuroplasticity" in their publications, and their peers belittled them for promoting a fanciful notion. Yet they persisted, slowly overturning the doctrine of the unchanging brain. They showed that children are not always stuck with the mental abilities they are born with; that the damaged brain can often reorganize itself so that when one part fails, another can often substitute; that if brain cells die, they can at times be replaced; that many "circuits" and even basic reflexes that we think are hardwired are not [Preface].

Discovering the content presented by Doidge acted as a catapult into examining how and why the circumstances in my mom's life and in mine resulted in such drastically different outcomes. Throughout Mom's life her brain was being shaped unknowingly by the fear and sure terror of what she believed to be happening. Early in my childhood I witnessed my mom's behavior in reaction to her circumstances. Fortunately, as a child with a highly malleable brain, I could also simulate how a much different approach might be used. In *The Brain That Changes Itself*, Doidge explains how neuroplasticity can limit or expand what we are capable of, based on how it is cultivated.

> Human plasticity broadly understood, the elucidation of human neural plasticity in our time, if carefully thought through, shows that

plasticity is far too subtle a phenomenon to unambiguously support a more constrained or unconstrained view of human nature, because in fact it contributes to both human rigidity and flexibility, depending upon how it is cultivated [318].

Mom wasn't clinically symptomatic until she approached age 40 but what should have been a blessing quickly became a curse. Her siblings lived from 12 to 20 years after the first symptoms began. And keep in mind that the symptoms of this disease in the first five years of onset are in stark contrast to the symptoms in the last five years. Prior to dying from cerebellar degeneration, muscles that allow your lungs to breathe can no longer effectively maintain this function. Alternatively, the risk of choking increases due to muscles in the throat being unable to coordinate swallowing. My mom was the youngest of five and had lived through her four siblings' struggles. I did not fully discover the details of their experiences until my mid–40s. Until then I had not contemplated what had occurred or how this impacted her life.

SMALL TOWN

My childhood overflowed with joyful memories while growing up in rural northern Indiana in Warsaw. Before I was born, Mom and Dad helped design and Dad even helped put the shingles on our house in Southbrook Park. It had a uniquely "home" feel. Cushions were built into the floor around the fireplace, there was a "woodbox," a small opening in the side of the house allowed food to go from the kitchen directly outside to the pool area. There was a pulley system zipline that extended down the ravine in the back yard, a pinball machine and pool table in the basement and a treehouse that Dad built with a rope ladder entrance. Even though I didn't realize why at the time, I was crushed when I found out we would move across town when I was eight.

Scott was a year ahead of me in elementary school, and by the time we were in the third and fourth grades, Todd and Brian were in high school. We had a huge wooded area behind our house where Scott and I would often play and explore. We had a nearby creek filled with crawfish and we had plenty of other children in the neighborhood to play with. We would get together with our parents' friends and Dad's family on the weekends and almost always go to church on Sunday. Mom took care of the house, meals and organizing schedules for Scott and me. Mom would often listen to records of Loretta Lynn, Tammy Wynette, Dolly Parton, and Patsy Cline. Dad naturally took the lead of reading to us each night. On weekends we sang songs like "Rocky Top" by John Denver and "Me & Bobby McGee" by Chris Kristofferson while he played guitar.

When Brian was in middle school, he and his friends formed a band, Fortress. I remember listening to them practice down in our basement. I still get nostalgic when I hear Journey's "Don't Stop Believing." It is the same basement where, when I was four, I ignorantly placed a hockey stick behind my head with my hands over each end of the stick. Then, either chasing toward or running away from something, I fell squarely on my face, my hands unable to break the fall. I ended up in the emergency room with a concussion.

My mom enjoyed playing the organ and doing puzzles, cerebral hobbies. My dad played basketball through college and I favored his preference for physical work that required mental

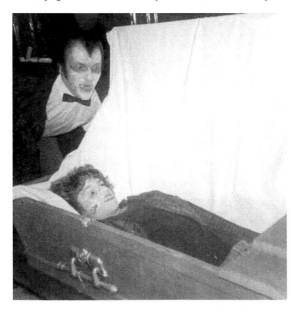

Robert Creighton leans over Todd Creighton in a coffin at a Halloween party at Otterbein Methodist Church, Atwood, Indiana, 1977.

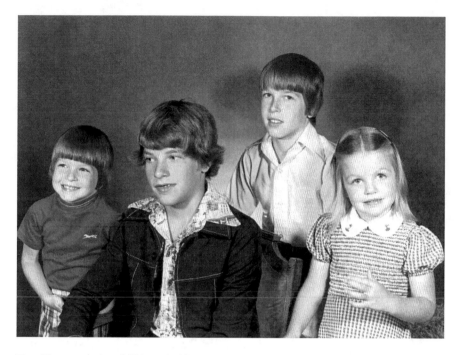

Family portrait of (from left) Scott, Todd, Brian and Dana Creighton in Warsaw, Indiana, 1977.

focus. When I was seven or eight my dad introduced Scott and me to how important keeping fit was to him. He took us on runs with him, at our pace, of course. I also distinctly remember my mom and dad stopping during the middle of any daily event and fully embracing each other in a prolonged hug. A conscious effort by each of them to take time to appreciate whatever the other had been doing for our whole family.

Dad was a biology teacher and Mom stayed at home so during summers we were all off together. When I was five, all six of us piled into our camper and for five weeks we drove across the country, visiting family on my dad's side in San Francisco. We stopped in Yellowstone and Glacier national parks, Mt. Rushmore and Salt Lake City. This stop in Utah included glider rides for everyone except Mom, who was terrified of the idea. I was over the moon to go visit the studio of the *Donny and Marie Show*, which I would watch with

Mom and Dad—unfortunately, it was closed the day we arrived, so we couldn't go in.

By the time I was six, Dad was going to the farm every day after he taught school to help his dad, Russell, with chores on the 125-acre farm. At this point, Grandpa only had beef cattle, but the work required keeping the 100-plus head of cattle fed with bales of hay through the winter months. New calves were born every spring and had to be sold when they grew to be 800 pounds. There was fixing miles of fence and responding to ailing cattle, among many other things. We spent a lot of time out at the farm, and it was not always sunshine and lemonade. Dad would take us out to his dad's farm and the four of us kids would help bale hay. Scott and I were much younger and smaller, so we lucked out of the most strenuous work. But then Dad also gave us "jobs" to do like picking up rocks in the field. We would tag along with him on weekends, which was always entertaining and educational, like when we would watch the calves get castrated.

Grandpa also had horses and he loved raising, breaking and teaching his grandchildren to ride and care for them. Grandpa had gotten rid of his horses that he had enjoyed for the previous five decades. But now approaching 80, he was finding it harder to keep up with all the farmland and the cattle. It was decided that we would move into the farmhouse and my dad would take over all the farming duties, in addition to teaching at the middle school.

We sold our house in Southbrook Park before my grandparents moved out of theirs, so we rented a house in Hersher's Addition in the same neighborhood that my parents lived in where all three boys were born. We could now walk to school and had many neighborhood friends from Washington Elementary School nearby. Mom, Dad, Scott and I were active in church activities and time was spent in the summer with other families from the church, including camping. Scott and I even took a road trip with the church youth group to see Jim and Tammy Faye Bakker tape their show *The PTL Club* ("PTL" meant "Praise the Lord") in Fort Mill, South Carolina.

———————————

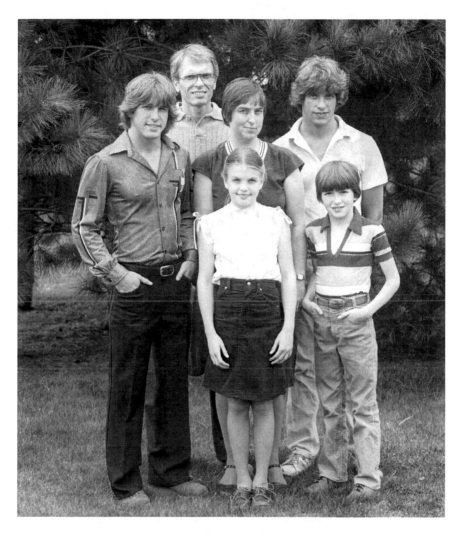

Family picture taken for our church: (back row from left) Brian, Robert, Marge, and Todd; Dana and Scott, for Atwood Otterbein Methodist Church, 1982.

In this rental house in December 1982, my dad, the biology teacher gave a lecture that he was dreading. He revealed to his four children what Mom's diagnosis was. He explained to us how a genetically dominant mutation was passed from parent to child, each time with a 50 percent chance of passing on the disease. I was 9, Scott

11, Brian 17, and Todd 20. My dad's explanation to us about these facts were interpreted and digested in wildly different ways. My childlike state of mind forced this information probably to the side somewhere that I certainly could never forget even if I had tried to. The gravity of this news was apparent from the obvious discomfort it caused my parents to utter their words.

Over the next year, Mom would often become very short-tempered with angry outbursts directed toward my dad. These were about common household issues, but the emotions attached to the circumstances were wildly exaggerated. For weeks, she would cry and moan when she went to bed each night, while she contemplated how this happened and how they could possibly manage this situation. I had recently started playing basketball and I totally immersed myself in playing for the next 15 years. My dad introduced me to the term "mental toughness" early in my life. This was not a single lesson but an ongoing dialogue he had with me through college. This lesson would not only apply to basketball but to many aspects of my life.

Mom was diagnosed when I was in the mid-point of my ninth year. Gradually, I began to see the two of us as more and more different. We of course shared similarities, like our appreciation for organization and planning, interior design and sweets. When we moved to my grandparents' farmhouse it was appropriately decorated in the style of the 1950s, when the house was built. I would join my mom to visit her friend Alma, an interior designer. I was in heaven looking through and helping choose from the swatches of wallpaper and carpet choices to update the farmhouse to the 1980s. During this timeframe, my mom had set horrible and tragic expectations for herself as she realized she was living her worst fears—a reality that already played out in front of her after the end of all her siblings' struggles with the same disease. And the real possibility that this had already been passed on to her children.

I, on the other hand, was blissfully ignorant of these circumstances. My mother did not speak freely about any of her family, many of whom were already deceased. Only her mom, Lorene, would make consistent but infrequent visits to our house and she would

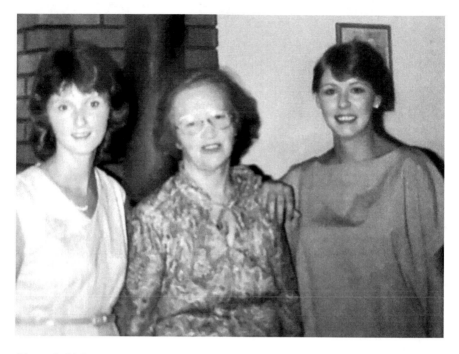

(From left) Betsy, Lorene and Marti Poynter at Granny's Main Street apartment in Kokomo, Indiana, 1982.

stay for a few days at a time. She didn't talk about other family members that I recall. I have memories of occasional visits from cousins Marti and, to a lesser extent, her younger sister Betsy, who was already in a wheelchair in her 20s. At the time I was not even aware that their mother Carolyn was my mother's sister. She had died from the family disease when I was one, in 1974.

HORNET, TIGER

Almost in parallel with Mom's diagnosis and continued downfall I clung to the game of basketball like my life depended on it. Fourth grade was my first year on the team for the Washington Hornets and I rarely played. I began attending Lady Tiger basketball camp that summer and started getting instruction from high school players.

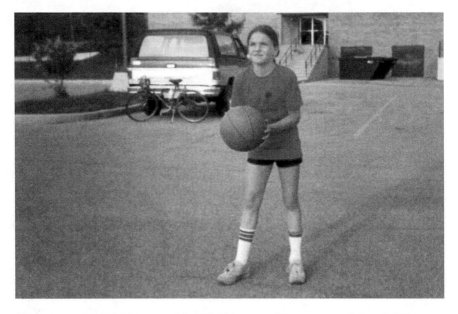

Dana practicing shots outside Washington Elementary School, Warsaw, Indiana, 1983.

They were dedicated and hardworking high school girls that I looked up to something fierce. I suddenly had the comradery of sisters who were helping me gain the skills I needed to become better instead of the three brothers I had who got enjoyment from making things difficult for me. When we lived in Southbrook Park, I broke out in tears when I came home and realized Todd and Brian had placed my beloved yellow bike with a banana seat and adorned with streamers high up in a tree.

While we were living in that house in Southbrook, Dad's hand-written journal started to record the mileage of his runs, starting in 1973. It turned into a daily entry of brief factual documentation of events of the day, related to Mom or any of the kids. I asked my dad if he could look in his journal to see if he could fact check if some of my early memories happened when I thought they did. Dad emailed me his journal entries that were documented by him in 1983. This was when I was nine years old and weeks after Mom's diagnosis. He sent me only the entries involving Mom or me.

Dad's Logbook

January 1983
15   Dana, Gymnastic Meet in Logansport.
19   Dana: Basketball game at Jefferson. Played 4 or 5 min.
22   Cancelled our trip to Indy weather icy.
29   Marge, depression returns.
30   Dana, Gymnastics meet, Laporte. Boyers went along.

February 1983
 9   Marge leave for Puerto Rico (with friend Colleen).
12   Dana Gymnastics meet, Chesterton.
18   Marge home from Puerto Rico 4 a.m.
23   Dana played Basketball vs Atwood. 1 point at FT line.
28   Dana BB tourney at Washington. 2 pts. on layup.

I have seen samples of my dad's journal for my whole life. Seeing it pasted into my own story makes me think of Jane Goodall, a stereotypical scientist at work documenting behaviors that would be used later to make some sort of sense out of the patterns observed. My dad had become accustomed to tough and unpleasant farm work throughout his childhood. Through that work he developed an intense work ethic. It would not only serve him well throughout his life, but it came in handy when he passed this trait to me. I also inherited his even keel, everything-is-under-control temperament.

The year my mom was diagnosed and for the next 15 years, I didn't talk with anyone about my family's predicament. That was our personal business, right? And what could anyone possibly do that would change anything? Without my noticing it then, my thoughts shifted away from Mom to myself. I was *not* focused on if I would be diagnosed someday, *but if I was, how would I react and live the rest of my life?* By the time I reached middle school my home life would start to shift and never be the same again For me, each morning was in fact a new day, and however unpleasant the previous day had been, this one could be different. I was dedicated to focusing on positive and affirming life goals, ignorant that there were more pressing issues to deal with.

I don't remember anything being drastically different right away but I remember bigger milestones over the next year or two:

I remember when Mom and Dad stopped going out to eat together; when my mom taught me and my brother how to do our own laundry; when Mom would go on family camping trips and stay in the camper; when she stopped coming on camping trips with us. My parents still did their best to give us life experiences to remember, but my mom was just no longer an active participant. When we planned a trip to Costa Rica when I was 14. Brian sprained his ankle badly when we were playing basketball in our backyard the day before we left. Dad and Todd carried him in a seat made by clasping their arms together through the jungle hikes. This was one of many times my dad exemplified how he chose to live, helping us squeeze all the juice out of every experience.

That next year was my first year in high school. I was invited to try out for the varsity basketball team. Letters of interest from colleges started streaming in during my sophomore year. I had received dozens of letters by my senior year and felt gratitude and sheer glee that I would get to choose which college I wanted to play for.

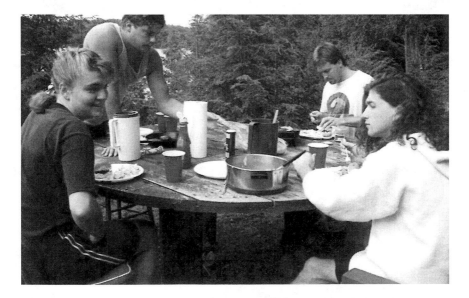

(From left) Dana, Todd, Brian and Scott on a family vacation at Chub Lake, Ontario, 1992.

My senior year I raked in most every top area player award and was selected to play for the Indiana All-Star Team with my best friend Liza. Early in my senior year I had visited the University of Toledo among a handful of other schools in the Midwest. I verbally committed to play basketball there. And I finally reached the pinnacle of my life so far—competing for a state championship at Market Square Arena in Indianapolis. We beat our opponent in the morning game and then faced Bedford North-Lawrence in the finals that afternoon. More than 15,000 fans packed the arena for the championship game. It was a hard-fought game between two teams with contrasting styles. Warsaw had the "twin towers," Liza and me, while Bedford relied on their two pint-sized but lightning-quick guards. Bedford had lost on this very stage the previous year. This year they would finally get their championship. I had dreamed and talked about winning a state championship since elementary school. I was devastated.

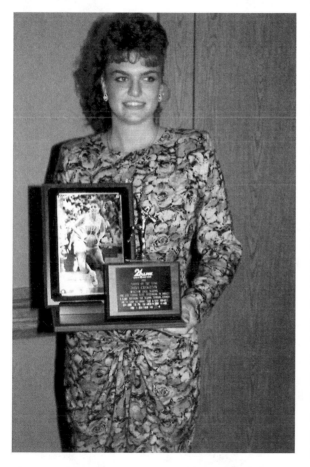

Dana Creighton receiving 21 Alive Fort Wayne Area Player of Year, Fort Wayne, Indiana, 1991.

Hoosier, Rocket

Since I had already decided to play for the Toledo Rockets, I wanted to cancel my upcoming visit to Indiana University (IU). My parents reminded me that I had already made a commitment to go, so I did. After visiting Bloomington in the spring as a senior in high school, I signed a letter of intent to play basketball for the Hoosiers the next fall. I loved the big, beautiful campus in southern Indiana and my newfound freedom. I made new friends in my dorm and I even had a couple of high school friends living in the same quad.

Soon after arriving on campus we began our preseason training. I struggled to get into a high level of fitness, and weight training with a strength training coach was new to me. Weeks later we started official practice and then games. I was used to being one of the tallest and strongest players in high school. Now I was one of the smallest forwards on my team and in the Big Ten. The fun-loving and charming head coach that had come to my house for a home visit the year before appeared to be a different person.

Early in the season he informed me that I wasn't consistently catching the ball. He suggested one of the assistant coaches work extra with me after practice. I did this wholeheartedly, wanting to do anything to get some more playing time. I got used to the bench more as the season progressed. Looking back, I find it hard to believe that one of the primary fundamental skills that I mastered in elementary school was haunting me as a college freshman.

It never occurred to me in the moment that my inability to consistently catch a ball might have been an early sign of what was in store for me. Or maybe the intensity level of the Big Ten was increasing my anxiety, causing the slightest of symptoms to escalate. I wasn't consciously aware of this at that time but I'm sure that his strategy to "fix" his perception of my weakness was the final straw that led to my departure from IU to the University of Toledo in Ohio.

I transferred to be a Rocket. Toledo thankfully was still interested in me after I had turned down their initial offer. During my redshirt year, I was beginning to gain the confidence I had lost during my freshman year as a Hoosier. I knew immediately that my major would be exercise science as I had taken an introductory class at IU. I started the coursework at Toledo and enjoyed the core classes and professors. The introduction to exercise science class I had taken in Bloomington would come in handy. The summer before my first year at Toledo I quickly got myself in great shape. Using interval training, I came to campus in good shape which gave me a physical as well as a mental edge. My redshirt year I had learned to get fulfillment from just being in practice since I couldn't play in games. I was thriving and was seriously enjoying being the fictitious star player for the upcoming opponents' teams.

In stark contrast, my home life was a tragic non-fiction, unfolding outside of my control. The last time I saw my mother alive was September 18, 1993. I was about to leave for college for the third fall in a row. I had taken this opportunity to give my mom a big hug and say "I love you" at the end of another summer spent at home. I know it doesn't sound like it should be an isolated incident for a mother and daughter, but it was in our case. I had always known my mother loved me, but she was just unable to show it. On this day, I was going off to college only one state away but would inevitably end up at home soon for the weekend.

It's odd. I didn't notice any difference in Mom's behavior or actions. When I said good-bye, she was sitting in her recliner, and as I went in for the hug, she accepted it but didn't fully embrace me as I wished she would. But this was her usual reaction when I would stage my annual farewell by professing my love for her on the day that I left for school each fall. I was pleased with myself for sneaking in my affection and then I looked forward to what this next year had in store. I made my three-hour drive across northern Indiana to Toledo in northwest Ohio. I spent the rest of the weekend settling back into my apartment and preparing for the first day of classes. Since I had already completed my redshirt year, I was really looking forward to finally being able to play in games.

On the morning of Monday, September 20, 1993, we were scheduled to have our team pictures taken. I was getting ready in my off-campus apartment that I shared with my teammate and friend from northwest Indiana. My dad called me to tell me my mother had taken her life. She had made a plan that would prove to be effective yet not risk my dad finding out until the next morning. He found her body in the running car in the closed garage. Out of all the scenarios I had devised that would lead to the last day of her life, this was never one of them. I don't remember many details of the next few hours, but I do remember that I cried the entire drive home and hearing a James Taylor song on the car radio, "Fire and Rain," only made me sob harder.

Upon hearing this news from my dad, I had many questions, but there was one question I didn't have, and that was *why*. I knew *why* she killed herself. But why couldn't she allow herself to be close to me? Was it too awful to fathom that she might have passed this condition to us kids? Our family had not talked freely about my mom's disease while she was alive. After her death, we certainly did not discuss it. I packaged up my pain neatly with a nice bow, to be opened later.

TIME MACHINE

The two summers prior to my mom's death, I had spent at home in Warsaw. My dad spent a lot of time overseeing the construction of their retirement cabin in Brown County, Indiana. I usually slept on the couch in the family room instead of in my upstairs bedroom. This way I could help my mom when she rolled down the hallway in her wheelchair from her bedroom each morning. That first night I was home after her death, I found myself sleeping on the same couch. I remember waking up in the morning to what I thought was the sound of my mom wheeling down the hall, which was so ingrained in my memory that it tricked my conscious mind into thinking she had just gotten up and was coming to the kitchen. Then I realized what had just happened and that I was home to attend her funeral.

To this day the smell of a bouquet of flowers transports me back. I had a large extended family on my dad's side. His father was one of six children and Grandpa's siblings were beginning to fade away before I was 10. Funerals are designed to bring families and loved ones together to provide comfort to one another. But on the day of Mom's funeral, it was private—like she requested—so there was no comfort to be given by others, just our secret grieving.

Her death happened right as my first season at Toledo as an eligible player was about to begin. Needless to say, it didn't go well for me that year. After Mom's suicide it became an insurmountable task to acknowledge the pain I was feeling and attempt to understand where it was coming from. I was focused on *not* letting my circumstances affect me, and practice makes perfect, right? I was hiding a secret, playing a role I wished for. But most importantly, I was trying to keep the mystery from others in the same way my mother had done. This article was written at the very beginning of the next season—here is part of it.

> Toledo basketball coach jokingly called her "the machine."
> But there wasn't much for Dana Creighton to joke about a year ago and if any machine was involved, it was a time machine she had trouble escaping.
> "I believe that if you work your hardest and do your best, things will work out," said Creighton. If it's a simple matter of hard work Fennelly said no one should worry about Creighton being successful. "She's a machine," Fennelly said. "She never stops running, never stops working. Nobody questions how badly she wants to get it done. I think on every team there is somebody who everybody pulls a little extra for and I think Dana Creighton is that person on our team [Dave Hackenberg, "Rockets Counting on Creighton," *Toledo Blade*, Nov. 7, 1994].

At the bottom of this Xeroxed copy was a handwritten note from Coach Fennelly.

> Dana—
> This was a nice story about you. I've enclosed a couple of extra copies for you to send to family and friends. I'm really excited about what kind of year you'll have in 94–95. No one is pulling more for you than me!
> Coach F
> P.S. maybe your three-point play to start the season is a good omen!

Chapter I. What Comes Next

I'm sure this article was the only one of my college career that was solely about me. It definitely got saved in my large box of scrapbooks and loose photos. Maybe his belief in me gave me hope that this year would be different. As I continued to write, another character in my story emerged. I knew Dr. Gunnar Brolinson well as he had been our physician for the basketball team. He attended all home games and traveled with us on road trips. He was a D.O. and had used manual manipulation on me during my basketball days to straighten out some of my lower back issues and neck and shoulder tightness.

> **MDs** practice allpathic medicine, the classical form of medicine, focused on the diagnosis and treatment of human diseases.
>
> **DOs** practice osteopathic medicine which is centered around a more holistic view of medicine in which the focus is on seeing the patient as a "whole person" to reach a diagnosis, rather than treating the symptoms alone.
>
> The belief is that all parts of the body work together and influence each other. Osteopathic medicine also places emphasis on the prevention of disease. In medical school, there is specific training on osteopathic manipulative treatment (OMT), a hands-on approach to diagnosis and treatment as well as disease prevention.

Dr. Brolinson was a strong proponent of visualization and he had used a hollowed out "coin" on a string to demonstrate this to us as a team before one of our away games in the locker room. Each of us had our own and we were instructed to hold the string with only our index finger and thumb. You can move the direction of the attached coin with your mind through the impulses your mind imposes through your fingers. This really had a strong effect on me, demonstrating the impact your mind can have directly on your body. One of the most important tools I gained from basketball was to anticipate. It helped me excel in high school offensively and then through college defensively—the combined forces of using my brain to focus on what was likely to happen next along with learned skills I had been practicing for 15 years. This enabled me to provide my team with a change in momentum that I had created.

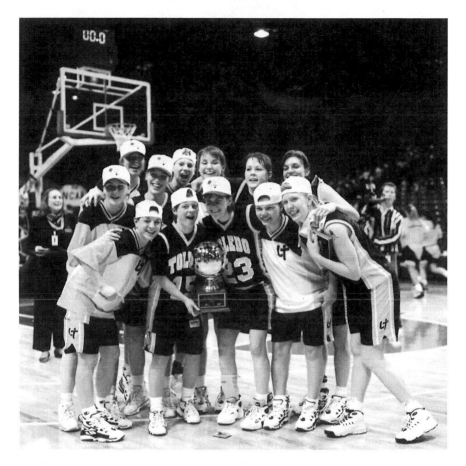

(Back row, from left) Gulsha Akkaya, Jennifer Holsclaw, Kim Knuth, Kim D'Angelo, Mimi Olsen, Trish Wagner and Dana Creighton with (front row, from left) Kristen Tews, Heather Smith, Denise Pickenpaugh, Leslie Favre and Angela Drake celebrating following MAC Championship win in Toledo, Ohio, 1996.

When I was a senior at Toledo, I remember a specific example of this happening. Whenever our opponent would score, I would take the ball and inbounds it to our point guard. As our firefly point guard Heather was dribbling up the floor, her defender was putting very tight pressure on her. After I ran past these two doing the tango, I decided to take advantage of the tenacious defense being applied. I placed myself squarely in line where Heather's defender would most certainly cross and covered my arms across my chest and awaited the blind-sided contact. It worked like a charm. Since I was set ahead of our contact, she technically initiated it and was called for the foul.

JUST FAKE IT

I completed my final basketball season and received my bachelor of science in exercise physiology. I decided to stay in Toledo and get a master's degree. There was an opportunity to vie for a graduate assistantship at Welltrack, the wellness program at Toledo Hospital. I had already completed my internship there for my undergraduate degree, so I knew the program manager, Christopher Miller. He had his Ph.D. in exercise physiology. He was good looking and knew how to have a blast, even at work. I got the assistantship and spent the next two years having an absolute scream with this new group of friends.

We would all strap on our rollerblades and wrist guards and head to the nearby paved pedestrian trail on campus which extended for 14 miles. We would road trip together to conferences and hang out with each other on weekends. Once we all drove to Michael's hometown in Michigan and went skiing on the lake. I also learned a hell of a lot and was studying physiology, biomechanics and nutrition along with testing and developing personalized exercise programs for hospital employees in the wellness center. I was serious about my studies for my master's degree and enjoyed graduate-level classes, including going to the cadaver lab to do a practical lab with doctoral students every week at the Medical College of Ohio.

However much relief I felt from not being tied down to the daily tedium of classes, practice, travel and games, I hadn't exactly acknowledged or appreciated the major distraction that basketball gave me. We were constantly preparing for new opponents, simulating their style of play during practice, with games every Wednesday and Saturday. During bus rides during the season, I studied and socialized. In the off season, our team would lift weights and run together.

While I was still in graduate school in Toledo in 1998, I reached out to our former team physician, Dr. Gunnar Brolinson. He was the director of Welltrack and I was technically working for him at the wellness center. I told him about my family's situation and he kindly referred me to Dr. Haynes Robinson, a geneticist at Toledo Hospital. After meeting with Dr. Robinson a few weeks later, he suggested that I request medical records from IU Medical Center in Indianapolis on Earl Poynter, my grandfather, or any of his family, as it related to an inherited cerebellar degeneration. I made the request, and I received several pages of records from my Grandpa Earl and his family. This was after my dad had already given me a copy of my mom's personal stash of records and letters the previous year. My mom's included her personal correspondence with doctors as well as letters within her family. These were stored in a folder and put away in a box in my closet.

This was two years into graduate school, and I had finished my coursework. Now it was time to complete my thesis, and I was sort of at a loss for what to do and how to do it. My favorite professor and advisor Dr. Fred Andres proposed a topic that I was enthusiastic about, all of it, including the development of the methods section, "Weight-Bearing Exercise and Markers of Bone Turnover in Female Athletes." In other words, it was about *the effects that different impact groups have on bone density compared in women's collegiate swimming, soccer and volleyball.* I was fortunate that Dr. Gunnar Brolinson would write a small grant and we received the funds to pay for the lab assays to measure bone turnover from urine and blood samples. It also covered the DEXA scans done at Toledo Hospital. I recruited my subjects, collected their various biological samples and ran the assays in the lab. I spent endless hours at the library searching for and making copies of references for the completion of my thesis and the paper we would publish based on the results.

Up until that point, I was wrapped up in my classes and working 20 hours a week, earning my assistantship. My mind didn't have a specific target to focus on and my life experiences up until then allowed me to avoid my circumstances and double up on the challenge that was visually in front of me. I did not keep an ongoing daily journal and never had. But when things got too overwhelming for me, I would write to release whatever was brewing inside me. I can't help but think that my dad's daily "journal" compelled me to "just write it down." By writing it down I had made an important step in claiming my feelings, even though it uncovered deep pain.

> August 9, 1999—Toledo, Ohio
>
> This is the worst I have felt for a long time. Not right now—I feel fine now. what is it? things bother me now that never used to bother me. I could always blow things off so easily. Now things just snowball. And I get so stubborn. I just want to start again and forget everything. It took me one beer to even write this. You have to decide in your own mind. Life is so miserable when you want it to be and so great when you make it great. All the little things that bother me usually boil down to one thing. I have no one right now. I feel like I don't have anyone right now…. People care about me—my family loves me. but that isn't enough right now…. I have to change my thinking and attitude.
>
> suck it up
> have some fun
> fake it!

Even though I was suffering a deep depression, Natalie Merchant was coming to play at the Toledo Zoo. This was a perfect opportunity to "fake it" since she was my all-time favorite singer. I remember it was cold outside and the zoo was still decorated for Christmas. Jane, who was our assistant basketball coach, drove with a few other former and current players. As the Ophelia concert went on, I began to feel incredibly joyful and happy singing out loud with everyone else. If you have ever seen Natalie perform, she is pure joy personified. She moves and dances in a way that is truly her own and she clearly has no qualms about expressing herself. I can remember listening to her album *Ophelia* in the summertime at the farmhouse. "Life Is Sweet" was my all-time favorite song. I depended on music as strongly as the sanctuary that I used to attend. I didn't realize this connection at the time, but I would continue to rely on music to pull me through trying times for the next 20 years.

One of these times was transitioning away from my somewhat predictable life spent on the court to not only a new job but one with a budding new business plan. Although I wasn't looking for a full-time job in Toledo, one found me. My advisor notified me of a job opportunity. A local pharmacy was starting a cardiopulmonary and exercise testing program and needed someone to travel with the testing equipment to different local clinics. I helped recruit doctors within the clinics to test their patients and provide results.

During this time, I had also developed a close friendship with Sophia, who had been the director of marketing for women's basketball while I played at Toledo. We both knew firsthand the deep wounds that loss can leave. I shared details about my family history, my grief and struggles that I had never shared with anyone before, including my well disguised unease about my chances of getting the family disease. She was the first person to see exactly who I was and not just the image of what appeared on the outside. We were more like soul sisters and she not only asked me hard questions but deeply listened to what I said. It was a relief to share my experiences with someone who actually spoke my language.

In my first job working for the pharmacy I was building business relationships, learning new software and testing protocols without the familiarity of anything I was used to. What I lacked in the technical aspects of cardiopulmonary testing I made up for in people skills. Mentally, physically, and emotionally it was exhausting. I would be so drained that I would take a nap nearly every day after work, then sleep all night. After a few months, the cardiopulmonary exercise testing business was slow going. The business plan was stagnating and so was my outlook.

CHAPTER II

Clinging to Hope

Write about the truth. If you write about the truth, somebody's living that. Not just somebody, there's a lot of people.—Loretta Lynn

SUBTLE INCONSISTENCY

Most of my life I only viewed my mom's circumstances as they happened in our immediate family and in my lifetime. It was like assuming you can predict a straight line with only one data point. More data points give you a better idea of where the line actually is. Fortunately, and unexpectedly, my immediate family had just reconnected with the handful of members of my mom's family in 2016. The information they provided would fuel a long, slow-burning fire I had been holding onto from an early age. For months, they provided answers to my questions. Keys that would unlock not just my mom's story but her whole family's story. I had just turned 43, yet the details of Mom's life remained buried in her history until I dredged them out.

My mom was the youngest of five and had four older siblings. Three of them had died by the time I was three, and the fourth died in 1980, all from an inherited neurodegenerative disease. Bob, the oldest, was 38 when he died, and his funeral was in 1969, before I was born. Carolyn was 39 and her funeral was in 1974, when I was one. Bill was 44 and his funeral was in 1976. I was three and we did not go to his funeral. The last funeral, for David Lee, who was 46 in 1980, took place when I was six, turning seven that year. The first memories I have of attending a funeral on Mom's side were around age seven. I knew it must be on my mom's side since I didn't know anyone or even whose funeral it was. I was in the dark about most everything about her family.

Since I didn't have the information, I made up my own story. In my mind, I was attending my grandfather's funeral—except he died in 1975, when I was two. Until recently, when I found out otherwise, I would have told you that I had memories of my mom's father, Earl. When we would visit their apartment in Kokomo, he was in a wheelchair and he never talked to me. Grandma didn't move into an apartment until after Grandpa's death. Her last living son, David Lee, who was in a wheelchair, moved in with her. I distinctly remember a lot from when I was nine years old, in 1982. This was the year that my mom at age 42 was finally diagnosed with the same condition that had already killed all four of her siblings.

How it was able to steadily destroy her hope involved a series of events that began in the late 1950s, in mom's late teen years. Her older brothers Bob and Bill suffered from a similar neurological condition and were eventually given the diagnosis of Friedreich's Ataxia (FA). Mom's older sister Carolyn was then diagnosed with FA in her early 20s when she was living in Texas. Clinicians across the country were doing the best they could to identify what they were seeing, but they were also following the lead and taking cues from each other. This was taken directly from Carolyn's medical record at IU Medical Center just weeks before her death.

> Carolyn (Poynter) Thomas June 12, 1974
>
> This 39-year-old white woman was admitted to University Hospital for treatment of a chronic progressive neurologic disorder which has been diagnosed as Friedreich's Ataxia. There have been multiple affected individuals in the family and a pattern that is consistent with autosomal dominant inheritance...
>
> Impression: ...dominantly inherited progressive neurologic degenerative disease...
>
> Comment: There are several inherited neurological disorders associated with abnormalities of movement... [Walter Nance, M.D.].

The statement at the top—this condition has been "diagnosed as Friedreich's Ataxia" and the next—it "is consistent with autosomal dominant inheritance"—are contradictions of each other. Friedreich's Ataxia (FA) was described in 1863 by Nikolaus Friedreich, a professor of medicine in Heidelberg, Germany. He described how it is recessively inherited. Surely no one in my mom's family even picked up on this inconsistency. It had already easily slipped past the clinicians.

This was the most common form of Ataxia, so likely doctors just labeled it as such because it was the closest thing that matched based on the symptoms being presented, along with age of onset (20s), which was a factor that led clinicians to assume they were on the right track. Since the family's symptoms appeared to mostly match, it was FA until proven otherwise. But in 1971, doctors at the Mayo Clinic gave my mom their opinion that they were not certain FA was even the correct diagnosis—and it was not.

Misdirection

When you stop and ask for directions, you are assuming that the other person (a) knows where you want to go and (b) will be able to effectively articulate those instructions to you in a way that will be understood. Some people would explain that even stopping to ask a stranger for directions means you have already reached a threshold of desperation. Some people may misinterpret where your destination is. Or even doing the best they can, some just may get you going in a general direction of where they think you might want to go. Sometimes communication between doctors and patients can have similar breakdowns that can go in both directions.

The doctors saw wide differences in the range of age of onset in Mom's family. My grandma Lorene reported in 1964 that her husband's father, Willie, and his brother Ralph both had Parkinson's disease. Since their symptoms were not established until later in life, the diagnosis of Parkinson's was given to them. Then it was noted in the medical record in 1974 that Earl had Friedreich's Ataxia (since four of five of his children were symptomatic or deceased because of it). Looking at all of this now, it was easy to see how doctors doing the best they could with the information they had available to them had been inadvertently misdirecting the family by diagnosing the same condition with different names.

To hopefully reduce that variability, Mom and Dad specifically went to the Mayo Clinic in Minneapolis, Minnesota, the place that had earned the distinction of having the most highly trained and knowledgeable doctors. On December 30, 1970, Dad writes a letter to "genetic counseling services" at Mayo. He addresses the letter "Gentlemen." As he explains, Mom and Dad already had Todd (eight) and Brian (six) and she was eight weeks pregnant. The letter states that multiple family members have fallen victim to Friedreich's Ataxia. Written between the lines: *we are looking for some guidance that everything will be all right.*

I have reproduced the letter here though the quality of the original is poor.

> 204 Tyner Dr.
> Warsaw, Indiana 46580
> December 30, 1970
>
> Genetic Counseling Service
> Mayo Clinic
> Rochester, Minn. 55901
>
> Gentlemen:
>
> I would like some information concerning whether or not genetic counseling service can be obtained by correspondence or if a visit to the clinic is necessary? Perhaps more information can help you determine this.
>
> Several members of my wife's family have gradually become victims of Friedreich's ataxia (her father, three brothers and one sister).
>
> My wife and I have two sons (ages 8 and 6) who were born just prior to the time when the ataxia in my wife's family was first being diagnosed. We planned no more children. Mainly because of the hereditary question of which we knew very little.
>
> However, my wife is now eight weeks pregnant and we are very concerned about the hereditary condition of the unborn. Cannot

be predicted what will be the risk for wife and our two sons being affected and now our unborn. Can anything be done in any of the circumstances?

We can supply further information including reports from my wife's father, Dr. autopsy reports on the deceased and other information. You may call us collect in Warsaw, Indiana (219) 267-6551.

Sincerely,
Robert Creighton

Dad received Dr. Hymie Gordon's reply to him stating genetic counseling could only be provided in person.

I have doubts about diagnosis of FA—he refers to FA unsteadiness is well established in 20s—your wife's family seems to have had a much later onset.

This "doubt" was translated by my mom as hope that things may not be as bad as she thought.

Assuring Mom and Dad that everything possible was being done, he both adamantly and confidently conveyed via correspondence that he could step in and mediate this uncertainty. Dr. Gordon responded "colleagues in neurology are expert in the ataxic group of diseases and would add to precision of genetic counseling...."

Mom and Dad flew to the Mayo Clinic and neurologist Dr. Peter Dyck examined Mom and determined she was asymptomatic. At the time, there was not a definitive genetic test available and "risk assessments" were based on the neurologist's confidence in the clinical examination. Even when there were no clear signs of degeneration on examination, there remained some possibility that symptoms could develop in the future. Then, miraculously, her chances were drastically reduced. Dr. Hymie Gordon reported, "you have about a 10 percent chance of having this same condition." Ten percent, not 50.

Both my mom and dad were college educated, and my dad had a master's degree in biology. This "10 percent chance" was a little like a magician using smoke and mirrors to distract the audience from what might be happening. It probably did not take much to convince my parents, who came there looking for answers but would happily walk away with hope that their outlook would be different than the rest of Mom's family. What possible good could come from telling my mom, an asymptomatic pregnant 31-year-old mother of two, that her chances were still 50 percent of showing symptoms in her lifetime? Dr. Hymie Gordon did not have any treatment options to provide my mom or a precise diagnosis. And he was the chair of medical genetics, not a neurologist. Clinically nothing had changed Mom's chances of becoming affected too.

Except for the hope and maybe even sheer fantasy that everything would work out OK this time around. That saving her mental anguish that was surely haunting her could buy a few more productive years with her growing family. This allowed my mom to cling to hope, when that's what Dr. Hymie Gordon offered to her. She held the doctor's opinion so high because she was clearly so close to the personal side of being a mother. She needed to consider her and my dad's desires only within the context of clinical evaluation and input. The medical opinion was of paramount importance to her and my dad's family planning. She and my dad were, however, making major life decisions on what they were being told. The different clinicians who were spread across different institutions were taking the information of previous reports. In studying all of Mom's records, including records about her siblings, I discovered how differently this disease was perceived by both clinicians and patients.

From a clinical perspective, they were making their best guesses considering the symptoms they saw that seemed to fit with Friedreich's Ataxia, which was the most common form of this type of hereditary disease. Clinicians referred to the condition to my parents as Poynter Disease. This term was coined as the doctors at Mayo referred to it in 1971, when my parents made their visit there. This was a personalized name given to the condition responsible for the symptoms that by then had the neurologists in their own frenzied state. This changing terminology was a signal to my mom that they were taking stabs in the dark.

From a patient's perspective, they were passing any information on to other family members as they were being given it. My mom and her siblings were shaping their own version of their reality while juggling the differing medical jargon flying around that was unfamiliar to them. As slowly as it became clearer clinically as time went on, this disease remained nebulous and haunting for my mother's entire adult life. An overly inflated prognosis that was well meaning was also in conflict with her own reality. Since the mid–1960s my mom had been struggling with her inner self who was hypersensitive to her own movements pitted against what the doctors now had just told her had little chance of ever happening.

Ultimately it didn't matter what they called it—it was a dominantly inherited cerebellar degeneration that could be passed on to 50 percent of the offspring of the affected person. That information was clear and consistent in the medical records of Mom's siblings Bill and Carolyn. And this information trickled down to my mom. Even though she had not shown any signs or symptoms, she should have fallen into this category too. That is, until she came to the Mayo Clinic in late January of 1971 and was given a reduced chance, now a 10 percent chance of getting it, not 50.

The information my mom was given was clearly spun in a way that would appease her in her "situation." She was told "now you are asymptomatic" and "there is about a 10 percent chance of your getting it." What my parents thought they were asking for and getting was a sound and reliable clinical opinion they could use to evaluate my mom's current risk and the future risk for her children. Technically, Mom and Dad were seeking and received from Hymie Gordon a "genetic counseling recommendation" or a green light to go ahead living the life they already started and not allow the possibility of this diagnosis to guide those decisions. Having thought she was at 50 percent risk before coming to the Mayo Clinic and now having it go down to 10 percent, she joyfully prepared for having a third child join the family. Scott was born in August of 1971 and then I came along in April of 1973.

CONFLICT OF INTEREST

> A widely used definition is: "A conflict of interest is a set of circumstances that creates a risk that professional judgement or actions regarding a primary interest will be unduly influenced by a secondary interest." *Primary interest* refers to the principal goals of the profession or activity, such as the protection of clients, the health of patients, the integrity of research, and the duties of public officer.—Wikipedia

It was not an issue that Dr. Hymie Gordon had just been appointed chair of the department of medical genetics at the Mayo Clinic in 1969 or that he had just immigrated to the United States a year before seeing my mom. It may have been an issue that he was a staunch "right to life" proponent. This was his right to have his own beliefs, one way or another. But did it influence the recommendations he gave to patients as chair of medical genetics at the Mayo Clinic? Randy Alcorn wrote in "Scientists Attest to Life Beginning at Conception" on March 18, 2010,

> A United States Senate Judiciary Subcommittee invited experts to testify on the question of when life begins. All of the quotes from the following experts come directly from the official government record of their testimony.[1]
>   Professor Hymie Gordon, Mayo Clinic: "By all the criteria of modern molecular biology, life is present from the moment of conception."
>   1 Report, Subcommittee on Separation of Powers to Senate Judiciary Committee S-158, 97th Congress, 1st Session 1981.

Timothy Oliver wrote on February 9, 2012, on the website of the National Association for the Advancement of Preborn Children,

> Perhaps Dr. Hymie Gordon, professor of medical genetics and a physician at the prestigious Mayo Clinic, best summarized the perspective of science when he said, "I think we can now also say that the question of the beginning of life—when life begins—is no longer a question for theological or philosophical dispute. It is an established scientific fact. Theologians and philosophers may go on to debate the meaning of life or purpose of life, but it is an established fact that all life, including human life, begins at the moment of conception."

Mom's chances of showing any symptoms in the future were still fifty percent, not ten. At first, my reaction to this was that without the use of a crystal ball this was what this doctor estimated her chances being, because she was not showing symptoms currently and she was already thirty-one. It was certainly not out of the question that mom might exhibit symptoms after age thirty. After my mom was given her reduced risk, she held on for dear life to the hope that our family would be spared the horrors of this condition. She did not have the option of having genetic testing done. The genetic marker linked to this mutation wasn't discovered until 1996, when it was identified as Spinocerebellar Ataxia Type 2 (SCA2). In *The Inheritance*, Julie had already witnessed her mother and sisters slip away into the depths of dementia. She was ready to find out which fifty percent chance her DNA would place her in. She compared getting her own test results back to being offered an oxygen mask.

> All she could think of was there had to be some reason for the pain, some insight. She struggled to articulate why knowing her mutation status would change that feeling, but her genetic counselor was able to explain "You are in a suspended state of life. You can't hold on to your past and everything you know from your past because you don't know your future. Your future is suspended. And my guess is you will feel differently after you know."
> Julie believes now that some of what he told her was standard operating procedure genetic counseling; but when he said "it was like someone put an oxygen mask on me." On June 19, 2003 her results came back: she was negative [*The Inheritance*, p118].

I have the luxury of compiling all this information and piecing it together after the fact. I'm aware that what happens in the moment clinically is sometimes a crapshoot. And that clinicians in the 60s, 70s and 80s had a fraction of the information they needed to confirm a diagnosis and then make recommendations based on them. The same neurologist, Dr. Peter Dyck, that had seen my mom and dad, saw Mom's brother Bill just days later in early February 1971. He was 39 and had been progressing for 15 years. Bill was told by Dr. Dyck that as an affected person, his own offspring would have a 50 percent chance of having the same condition. He gave Bill the diagnosis of dominantly inherited cerebellar Ataxia.

In contrast, my asymptomatic 31-year-old mother was told she had a 10 percent chance that she might develop symptoms in the future. And the fact that my mom was seen for a "genetic counseling" visit and Bill was being seen as a "clinical" visit might explain why different information was presented to each person. Dr. Hymie Gordon, chair of medical genetics, was most certainly not involved in Bill's clinical visit. Dr. Dyck was "consulted" but Mom likely interacted mostly with Dr. Gordon.

There was no new information. Bill and Marge shared a family history of this disease and both had a 50 percent chance of being affected. Bill had been showing symptoms since his mid–20s. He was also told that 50 percent of his offspring would be expected to get it and "sometimes mild involvement is not recognized and therefore some of their children will have the disorder" (eerily similar to my mom's actual circumstance). So why wasn't my mother given a similar explanation? She saw the same neurologist days prior to Bill's visit.

Clinicians at the Mayo Clinic did in fact clearly declare to Bill the nature of this disease as well as the inheritance pattern and did in fact significantly alter this same information when it was given to my mom. Unfortunately, my mom was the recipient of an overly hopeful prognosis by a clinician who decided that he needed to play the role of God—maybe for the sake of the unborn or maybe for the sake of my mom. And like all humans, she utilized the information she had been given to not only inform her choices but integrate that information into the story she told herself.

I came to understand how powerful this vocabulary was to patients and how much of a moving target it appeared to be for clinicians. What did get conveyed clearly to my mom was the clinician's *absolute uncertainty* about what was happening. But it only mattered to my mom that there was hope that her life would not turn out just like her siblings'. And this palpable uncertainty is what my mom held onto. For the next 10 years after she was given a 10 percent chance in 1971, she tried to resist her instinct that something was off. She had taken every precaution that she could have possibly imagined and jumped through every hoop which had led to her conclusion, based on all the evidence, to not let this disease or her own risk stop her from living the life she was already building and living. And that is what she tried to do.

Within Normal Limits

The roller coaster ride that my mother was on in 1971 does not end, but it rattles on to the next clinician who senses my mom's anxiety and urgency in 1980 and translates this into her own story about what is happening. Meanwhile, Mom's only sister, last two brothers and father all died between 1974 and 1980. My mom knew firsthand the wide clinical variability in medical diagnosis in her family. Multiple diagnoses were given to the same condition across various institutions. She went to Caylor-Nickel Research Foundation in Bluffton, Indiana, in 1980. My mom was seen on September 5, 1980, about her possible inheritance of cerebellar degeneration. The physical exam was performed by neurologist Dr. John Bossard, and Dr. Patricia Bader, director of clinical research, reviewed her history and concluded that Mom needed to be reassured that she was in fact *not* showing symptoms, even though Dr. Bader wrote,

> Recently [Marge] has become alarmed over isolated incidents of *staggering and poor coordination.* It is our opinion that Marge is not exhibiting early signs of this disease. We feel that the visit served to relieve much of her anxiety.

The neurologist reported testing was "within normal limits." Dr. Bader then gave a report that made sense in line with the neurologist's report. Dr. Bader concluded that Mom's reported "staggering and poor coordination" were due to her "heightened state of anxiety about having the condition." Then Mom returns again two years later reporting that she feels that symptoms have further progressed since her last visit. Dr. Bader documented,

I examined Mrs. Creighton in 1980 and was concerned that her voice was someone harsh, that she showed some difficulty in walking a straight line and hopping. I asked her to see Dr. John Bossard who felt that her exam was within normal limits.

On Ms. Creighton's first visit (1980) I feel that many of her difficulties might have had an emotional overlay, simply because she had just reached age forty which was the age her father was diagnosed at.

Dr. Bader had somehow erroneously interpreted this. Or maybe my mom reported that "his symptoms began in middle age" but he was not diagnosed at age 40. Dr. Bader used this as her story why Mom's "emotional overlay" was the issue. Dr. Bader continued:

Mrs. Creighton returned home and during the next two years noticed some progression of her difficulties. On physical exam in 1982, again, Dr. Patricia Bader noted some left sided weakness, some dyspraxia of speech, problems with finger to nose test, and she again however showed very poor ability to walk a straight line and she cannot hop at all.

I referred her to Dr. Stanley Whisman, and he feels that she has a positive neurological examination.

Mom tried to remain hopeful and she wrote a letter to her nephew Rick and niece Vickie that her case would likely be less severe than her siblings'. Mom told them not to panic if diagnosed. Since they were already in their 20s, she assured them their case would not be as severe as their cousin's disease. She told them,

I must have had it when I was thirty and am still walking at forty-three.... The thing that doctors kept telling me was that I would be expected to have a case similar to others in *my* generation.... I must warn you though that the doctors can't give definite answers because they don't know.... Prior to 1971 it was Friedreich's, when I went to Mayo in 1971, they called it Poynter Disease because each family had symptoms that were unique.... IU Med Center 1974 stated in Carolyn's medical record Friedreich's.... In 1982 in Bluffton, IN, doctor diagnosed me with Olivo-Ponto Cerebellar Atrophy (OPCA) type IV.... Again, don't panic. There are sometimes that I have difficulty believing that anything is wrong with me. Write if you have any more questions.

It was not likely for some of the family members to have Friedreich's and others to have something else. It would be inherited by everyone in the same family as the same condition. But Mom's age of onset was well beyond her 20s, when three of her four siblings succumbed. Then, by the mid–1960s, all four of Mom's siblings had symptoms of the disease, and clinicians were noting that this was a dominantly inherited condition. Earl died in 1975 of a heart attack but in 1974 he was given a new "probable" diagnosis, Olivo-Ponto Cerebellar Atrophy (OPCA), since that corresponded to a genetically dominant condition.

So this is the diagnosis my mom was given in November 1982. This just exemplifies that the clinicians were not immune to taking information and creating a story to tell the patient to make sense of the information presented. Her hope diminished as steadily as her fear escalated out of control. And I truly believe that in her gut she sensed that something had gone awry. Someone was at fault and to blame for how things panned out and she concluded that someone was herself. Mark Wolynn, author of *It Didn't Start with You*, gives this chilling recollection of how his sudden vision loss manifested the fear within him.

> The doctors were unable to tell me what caused my vision loss and what would heal it. Everything I tried on my own—vitamins, juice, fasts, hands-on healing—all seemed to make things worse. I was flummoxed. My greatest fear was unfolding in front of me and I was helpless to do anything about it. Blind, unable to take care of myself, and all alone, I would fall apart. My life would be ruined. I'd lose my will to live.
>
> I replayed the scenario over and over in my head. The more I thought about it, the deeper the hopeless feelings embedded in my body. I was sinking into sludge. Each time I tried to dig myself out, my thoughts go back to images of being all alone, helpless, and ruined. What I didn't know then was that the very words alone, helpless, and ruined were part of my personal language of fear. Unbridled and unrestrained they reeled in my head and rattled my body [3].

Unfortunately for my mom and my dad doctors now were loud and clear. You are in fact showing signs of this condition and you may have already passed it to your children. After her positive diagnosis in Bluffton she was blindsided and at the same time skeptical of each doctor's constantly changing story. With doubts still firmly in place, in May 1983, six months after her diagnosis of OPCA in Bluffton, Indiana, my mom traveled to the Mayo Clinic again hoping that Dr. Peter Dyck might provide her more hope. After examining her, he was now certain that she was, in fact, showing symptoms of cerebellar degeneration. On May 17, 1983, Dr. Dyck wrote a letter to Mom's local PCP in Warsaw, Indiana. Here is the last part.

> In summary, it is now apparent that Mrs. Creighton does have a dominantly inherited spinocerebellar degeneration. Clearly this is not FA because it is dominantly inherited, and it is not pure Olivoponto-cerebellar degeneration because there is evidence of involvement of the peripheral sensory system. I know that it must be very distressing for Mrs. Creighton as she was seen here eleven years ago, and the diagnosis was not made at that time.
>
> My assumption is that the symptomatic involvement has developed since that time ... the fact that she has late onset is clearly in her favor. I have discussed a program of physical fitness with her, emphasizing the need to keep her weight down.
>
> I have also encouraged her to continue going out and carrying on with the important functions she has as a mother and wife. I believe she tends to blame herself unnecessarily, particularly as it relates to her having children who are at risk for the disorder.

That was a conversation that unfortunately didn't carry much weight with my mom in 1983. It seems realistic and practical to expect that a patient could follow the wise advice offered by a doctor. But after putting together my rendition of her story, I wonder what impact that conversation might have had on her mind had it happened in 1971. If the seeds of hope might have taken root in her mind just as easily as the seeds of fear had. If talking about the realities of unfortunate possibilities had happened, as opposed to the genetic counseling information that she was given to distract her from proposing this very real possibility.

WILDFLOWERS

My own thoughts about what my mom must have gone through emotionally have greatly evolved over the years. Hers was a much different experience than mine, although we shared the same neurologic condition. We were both physically affected by Ataxia between our third and fourth decade. Only now can I begin to comprehend how the effects of my mom's condition and mine could have been more different. Here is *my own rendition* of what was going on in my mom's mind.

1965
I have a loving husband and we have two young boys. My three older siblings are being affected with something terrible. Am I at risk? And what about my two children?

1966–1968
All four of my siblings now have this condition, and my father. What is happening?

1969
My oldest brother Bob dies. I didn't even realize that I might be at risk until after I already had Todd and Brian, which would mean if I was diagnosed, I might have already passed this on to my two children. No more kids.

1970–1973
I am pregnant with my third. I am asymptomatic, and now I have been given a 10 percent chance of getting it—I have two more children born in 1971 and in 1973.

1971–1979
I am in conflict in living the life that I want to have and living the life that I know that I may be hiding from ... meanwhile two siblings both die as well as my father.

1980–1981
My anxiety and fear are dialed up as I reported staggering and poor coordination and clinically had trouble walking in straight line and hopping—but they tell me no, these are not symptoms ... last brother dies.

1982
The same symptoms I reported in 1980 have progressed, and now they tell me—oh wait, yes, you do have the same condition as the rest of your family.

My family had just reconnected with our first cousins Marti, Vickie and Jeff in the spring of 2016. They were my mom's only living nieces and nephew. I had arranged this trip with Marti and Vickie, who were both born in 1958. This was 15 years before I was born and when my mom was only 18. Jeff, Marti and Vickie were all approaching 60 and not affected by Ataxia, but all three had a sibling as well as a parent who died from it. They drove down to visit my brothers Todd, Brian and me at my dad's cabin in southern Indiana. We had been Facebook friends for a few years, but it felt like it was time for a face to face. It was at this visit when I remember meeting Vickie for the first time. She reminded me that we had met once or twice when I was around eight. Vickie was the daughter of my mom's brother Bill. According to her, my mom and Bill got along great, which was a surprise to me as I knew nothing about their family.

Brian and Todd had limited memories of these three cousins from their childhood. Marti is the only cousin of these three that I have memories of, as my mom kept in contact with her after her sister Carolyn and Marti's mother died from the family disease in 1974. I have few but infrequent memories of Marti as a child. Much to my surprise, I found out that she and my mom had an especially close bond. Marti would stay with my parents for several days at a time leading up to and shortly after Todd was born in November 1962. Her mom Carolyn had recently been in a fiery car accident. Carolyn, who was already suffering from the family disease, spent close to a year in the hospital in 1963 recovering from her burns. They told Marti, only five years old, that her mom probably wouldn't make it. She did make it, for 11 more years.

After we had lunch at my dad's, we went to visit with Todd, just down the road. Listening to my brothers and cousins talk, I was having a hard time following their conversations. They were telling stories and rattling off names, most of which were foreign to me, as I would have not been born yet. They told a series of stories that resembled a plot from Bugs Bunny and Yosemite Sam. Like the time Vickie was holding her brother Mike's pet monkey, Candy. Something startled Candy and she freaked out and got tangled in Vickie's long hair. Within a family, there are stories some have to share that can unlock answers for others. It wasn't too long after this visit from my cousins that I began to really consider and contemplate how Mom felt her entire life, from her perspective and not mine.

When I got home to Durham, I called Vickie several times trying to recreate my childhood, but this time with all the information that was missing as I lived it. Vickie said that she and Marti would be making a trip to the two cemeteries where multiple family members were buried. She offered to take photos of the headstones so I would have birth and death dates to help me write it all out. A few weeks later she texted me photos of all the headstones of our deceased family buried near Kokomo. I wrote out the pedigree and then it became shockingly clear.

I saw on paper how my mom had seen all her siblings and father die during the same timeframe that she was building her own family with my dad. And how deeply ingrained in her psyche the devastation of this disease must have caused. Dad told me that my mom would rarely if ever talk about her family to him. Mom distanced herself from her own right to feel those losses but then further distanced herself by mindfully disassociating herself from her family. She limited their interactions because of the prejudices, drinking, promiscuity, and domestic abuse in members of her family, making it mentally easier for her to see our family as completely separate from hers.

By the time of her diagnosis in 1982, our first cousins were already being affected—my cousin Mike was symptomatic around age 12 and died in 1984 at the age of 31. Mike was Vickie's older brother and the son of my mom's brother Bill. He had been showing signs of the family disease since his mid–20s, in the 1950s. It would not be until 1996 that a genetic test would be available to test for a definitive positive or negative status. Since Mom died in 1993, no one in our family was under a neurologist's care. Had a test been available in 1970, my mom would have most certainly opted to know her status. And then I would have certainly never been born in 1973. When I was in college, I used to enjoy watching *The Joy of Painting*. Bob Ross was the host of this PBS show from 1983 to 1994 and he said this:

> As you paint, you'll see all kinds of things happening on your canvas. Very soon, you learn how to use all of these beautiful little things. We don't make mistakes we have happy accidents.

56

I can't help but feel like a "happy accident" too. Throughout my life, events would appear on my canvas and it would be up to me to create something beautiful from them. Several weeks after our initial visit at Dad's cabin, Vickie called me to tell me that she found some of my mom's memorabilia from her high school graduation that she wanted me to have. I told her just to hang on to it and that I would try to make a trip up to Kokomo in the fall. I had a growing number of questions for her. So in October 2017, I traveled to Indiana. This trip was made specifically to spend time talking with and connecting with the few remaining family members from my mom's side of the family, in Kokomo, north of Indianapolis. My older brother Brian picked me up from the airport and we headed straight up Highway 30.

When we arrived, there were dozens of photos of the Poynter family dating as far back as the early 1900s covering her kitchen table. In addition to Vickie, Marti and Jeff, there was also their niece Kara, my first cousin, once removed. As we all were around the table looking at and talking about the photos, I recognized a school picture of a probably 12-year-old girl that had been hanging on a huge bulletin board of pictures in our childhood home. I picked it up and asked, "Who is this?" Everyone pointed at Kara—I was dumbfounded. My mom had gotten Kara's school picture probably from my grandma and posted it to our family bulletin board around 1985.

I am certain she never told me who this was at the time as I was always curious about her family and would have remembered it if she did. I never did inquire directly because her family was something that she never talked about with us. We all just chatted about the pictures as we made up scenarios about what might have been happening while the photos were being taken.

My two oldest brothers have memories of visiting and playing with their cousins on Mom's side throughout the 1960s. And 1970 was right around the time when my mother made it a point to isolate herself and our family from hers. When I was born in 1973, Scott was one and a half, Brian was eight and Todd was 10. Since my mom was the youngest in her family, Scott and I didn't have any first cousins that were our age anyway. Kara and I were both born in 1973, so she would have been a perfectly age-matched local cousin, who was about an hour away. But by 1980 Mom had been successful in keeping what remained of her entire family safely away from ours.

And by then, all her siblings and father had died, so she chose to remove them from her story altogether. Kara's grandfather, my uncle David Lee Poynter, had the family disease and died on the first day of July in 1980 at the age of 46. This was the funeral I recalled attending when I was seven. It was my mom's older brother's funeral, and not my grandfather Earl's, as I had been telling myself. Five months after David Lee's funeral, his son David Jr. died in a motorcycle accident at age 27. David Jr. was Kara's dad and my mom's nephew.

I listened to stories about my aunt and uncles, grandparents and their siblings that I had never heard before. It was fascinating to hear these stories and try to patch them together with what little memories I had as well as the research I had been doing for the past year about this side of my family. I continued to listen and learn for the next couple of days of my trip. I came away with a much better understanding of my own family's story as it was witnessed from my cousin's eyes.

During a more recent visit back to Kokomo, Vickie and Marti took me to two of the graveyards nearby where many of our family members are buried. I couldn't help but think about my own mom's gravestone in Warsaw with the trio of wildflowers on it. I also thought of when I was in graduate school and went to visit my childhood friend Liza in Sierra Vista, Arizona. I unknowingly picked out my tattoo from a nature book of wildflowers—three wild geraniums that closely resembled those three flowers my dad had chosen to mark Mom's grave.

CHAPTER III

Wrestle with Despair

One can never understand what hope is really about unless one wrestles with despair. The same is true with faith. There has to be some serious doubt, otherwise faith becomes merely a dogmatic formula, an orthodoxy, a way of evading the complexity of life, rather than a way of engaging honestly with life.—Cornel West

CAROLINA ON MY MIND

Trish had been my basketball teammate and was going to physical therapy school across town at the Medical College of Ohio in Toledo. After she finished school she decided to move to Raleigh, North Carolina, near her older sister and family. We had driven there on spring break of our senior year, so I knew I liked the area. Winters in Toledo were long and gray, and after a challenging year working for the pharmacy, I was more than ready for a change, especially if it involved lots of sun and jobs in Research Triangle Park (RTP). I moved to Raleigh to a one-bedroom apartment near Trish without a job ahead of time. I took some part-time and contract positions and was patching together enough to get by. This journal entry was written shortly after my dad drove with me from Toledo to Raleigh in a U-Haul truck 20 years ago.

September 3, 1999—Raleigh, North Carolina

When I left Toledo two weeks ago, I couldn't believe how incredibly unemotional I was. I've been there for 7 years and nothing. Didn't feel choked up in the least for anyone. Look how close I was to Sophia and she was there in front of me sobbing I could not even muster a tear.

Is it that I am so relieved and ready to leave Toledo or that I have completely disengaged myself from any emotional relationships? It really kind of worries me.

I balled when I left IU after 1 yr. and when Sally moved away from Toledo. Why not now? I feel so calloused and I shouldn't. I'm 26 and life hasn't been so easy for me, yet I consider myself to be so lucky in many ways. I'm trying not to be like mom was. Fending off love and feeling. Thinking it will be easier for everyone like that.

I remember the feelings of doom and hopelessness that had seeped into every part of my life. I was uncomfortable in social settings and easily annoyed that no one around me could possibly understand. I didn't even recognize at the time how my own deeply rooted fears were clearly in the driver's seat.

> I don't *want* to, but I feel powerless. I can try to fake it for periods of time, but I always come back to myself. I am the only one I can truly count on. I have so much anger and pain that I can't trust anyone to share that with. I feel like I can only cause someone more pain and have nothing to offer anyone. Why would anyone want me? I'm so jealous of people that have no reservations or apprehension about anything. I wish I could just have normal thoughts.
>
> Most of my life I feared death. It scared me—not to live anymore. I never wanted to give up what I had or what I was looking forward to. When I think about death now it doesn't scare me, I'm indifferent. I could just lie down, not get up and have no qualms. I don't *want* to die I just don't know that I wouldn't fight it. I hated to fear the end, it was so terrifying. but it scares me too that I've changed my thinking so drastically. It wasn't a conscious effort.

Feeling powerless led to self-doubt and the sense that others could identify that I had nothing to offer. My feelings about death had moved dramatically yet it felt like a shift that was not bound to conscious thought.

> I have nice things, great family, great friends. Why don't I feel worthy of any of it? I hate to feel weak and out of control. I've gone through periods of good and bad in my life. When I look back, I didn't realize how awful it was seeing Mom agonize over her disease. Hearing her cry and moan at night and just having to ignore it and pretend everything was ok.

I'm so lucky to have the opportunities I have had in life why do I feel
so worthless? Like I had nothing? I know it is wrong but that's how I
feel. I know I don't have a job right now. No direction. But surely that
can't be the answer. Then everything will be okay. Fine if that's it. I
hope it is. I hope I figure it out before I get too deep in my own self-pity
that I ruined what I started. That would truly be a shame.

When I went to my doctor to discuss my depression and these
thoughts, I was relieved to find confirmation that the symptoms I
reported warranted medical intervention. Using an antidepressant
has never been for me a quick fix. During the first few years I was just
happy to feel a sense of normalcy in my life again. It certainly did not
take away old wounds or prevent new ones. Over time, I viewed it
as a tool that I utilized to put myself in the optimal position to overcome the inherent barriers in my life.

I began searching for a full-time position, ideally in research,
and one that was as fulfilling as doing my thesis had turned out to be.
I decided to reach out to a former classmate I knew from the wellness
center at Toledo Hospital. Erin and I were not especially social as the
majority in our co ed social group preferred to drink lots of alco-
hol. I had heard she was living nearby in Durham, and I called her.
She informed me that there was a research assistant position open at
the UNC School of Nursing for a children's health study. I was scour-
ing the *News and Observer*, Raleigh's paper. This position was being
recruited locally in the *Daily Tar Heel* at UNC, targeting students in
Chapel Hill, since the positions were temporary.

I interviewed and was hired by the UNC School of Nursing into
a full-time but temporary position in a study led by Dr. Joanne Har-
rell. Only a few months into my new position, the project manager
who had hired me for the study announced she was taking another
position on campus. I was encouraged to interview for it as I had
already shown a genuine loyalty to the success of the project. I interviewed for and got the full-time position and managed the study for
the next four years until the funding ran out.

Working for Joanne was a dream. It was truly a team effort,
including our statistician Kant, a charming and intelligent man who

would always bring us treats and stories from his latest international journey, and Bob, the easily agitated but very insightful exercise physiologist who would always add some pizzazz to our regularly scheduled meetings. Joanne's style, leadership and nursing approach really resonated with me. She disseminated the research information back to the parents of the children she was studying, which included their child's blood glucose value and body mass index.

Aggregated countywide data was distributed to local health departments, information that could help the communities which helped her gain the data she needed. This all required extra time from me, but I was happy to do it. I also learned from her that team meetings were important brainstorming missions. Not only would I be required to type up minutes of these discussions, but most importantly document the *ACTION ITEMS* from each discussion. What was the take-away that was discussed and who was *going to be held accountable* for completing this by the next meeting? If it wasn't documented, it didn't happen.

While I was working at the UNC School of Nursing, I met Julie. She was getting her undergraduate degree and had volunteered to help a doctoral student, collect some data for our study. I trained Julie in how to use a centrifuge to spin down the blood that she would be collecting. We had a connection from the beginning and shared our love of cheeseburgers at Wendy's in the hospital the day we met. It wasn't until a few weeks later that we realized we also shared the loss of our mother. Julie was 14 when she watched as her mother struggled and deteriorated for two years fighting lung cancer while her father was blatantly cheating on his wife and the entire family. I lost my mother when I was 20. She had taken her own life after fearing and dreading her own demise as well as her children's demise for the last 20 years.

I moved to Raleigh specifically to find a job in research. I am also my father's daughter and shared with all three of my brothers our "frugal" ways. I had volunteered for various research studies across the area since moving there not only because I knew from experience that finding eligible and willing participants was difficult, but also for the money that was earned with relative ease. And there were plenty to choose from with UNC in Chapel Hill, Duke in Durham, and Research Triangle Park within minutes of me.

I had moved from an apartment in Raleigh to Durham, which was just a few miles from campus, down Highway 54 into Chapel Hill. After a few months I had settled into Durham nicely and I bought a small house. After more than two years of trial and error in the workforce in my new state of North Carolina, I felt happy about my life. I had found a rewarding job, bought a house and acquired a puppy. Zoe, a black Lab, had found me as she was wandering along the highway while I was traveling for my job. Sharon also wandered into my life. I interviewed her for one of our open positions at the UNC School of Nursing. The job was not exactly what she was looking for, but I had found a lifelong friend.

THE JAMES JOYCE PUB

I met Sean in January 2002, a few days before the Super Bowl. I was with my temporary housemate, Sharon, whom I had recently met at an interview at UNC, along with my new neighbor Coleen and her friend Ben. Ben and I were friends too, though he was vocal to me that he was interested in being more. I was not someone that needed to be with a partner all the time. If I wasn't absolutely interested, I was glad to drop it. The four of us didn't intend to, but we ended up at an Irish pub in Durham.

Sean had been golfing that day with his buddies in Raleigh, and they converged on the James Joyce in downtown Durham so we both ended up there somewhat by chance. Sean was with a group of Canadian nurses who had gone to school together and then traveled to North Carolina, looking for work. Sean had found nursing jobs in several cities in the eastern part of the state and had only moved to Chapel Hill from Wilmington a few weeks earlier. We were both working for UNC–Chapel Hill, me at the School of Nursing and Sean at the hospital. We chatted and listened to the band who was playing 90s alternative rock and played a lot of the Cure, one of my favorite choices from my high school days.

I have always had a difficult time articulating who I was to others, especially men. But since I had been taking an antidepressant for more than a year now, communicating had gotten much easier. It didn't hurt that I had a couple of beers on board. We had a good chemistry and Sean wrote his number down and gave it to me. The next week, I called him, and we met for coffee when he was on his way to work the night shift at the hospital. A few days later, we took my two dogs for a walk on the trails at the Botanical Gardens in Chapel Hill. We quickly inserted ourselves into each other's lives and routines. He typically worked the night shift and I would pack him a lunch and drop it off at his apartment before he would go to work. We introduced each other to friends and families, and by the end of our first year together it was evident to me that aside from a firm compatibility, we shared similar values and strong family connections.

I was more than proactive about my own health as I sought out a neurologist demanding that I establish my own baseline. One of my mom's greatest struggles was that every time a different neurologist examined her, she was compared not against her own baseline but was instead deemed as "within normal limits." I didn't want to walk down the same or even a remotely similar path as my mom did if I could help it. In 2004, I was "clinically asymptomatic" which was no surprise to me. I was happy that now my own baseline had been established. I did, however, have a slight amount of unease that I felt so compelled to seek this out.

When I think about our first few years together, Sean and I were both happy to have found each other and really appreciated our similarities as well as our many differences. Very early on, we were open and honest about our past failures and future worries. He openly disclosed to me that he had been married briefly before he had relocated to Chapel Hill. I disclosed to him that I had a 50 percent chance of having a serious neurological condition. These were not game changers for either of us. I took my chances and he took his. We accepted each other as we were. He bought a house nearby

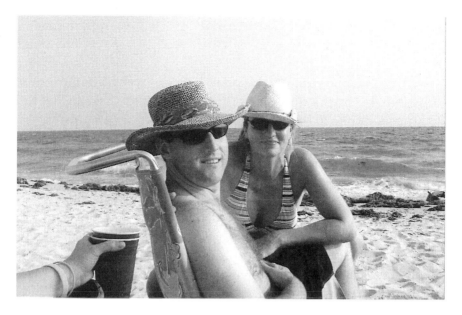

Sean and Dana celebrating the Fourth of July at Caswell Beach, North Carolina, 2003.

in Durham, but that arrangement only lasted about a year and then he just moved in with me. We prided ourselves on working together as a team as we renovated the bathroom, built a firepit in our backyard and cooked meals. We were building a life together that was not dependent on getting married—that is, until we started talking about starting a family.

We celebrated Canadian Thanksgiving the second Monday of October in 2005. We traveled to Calgary, Alberta, and stayed with Sean's aunt and uncle. Then Sean and I took a side trip to Banff and Lake Louise, less than two hours away. We went skiing in Banff—part of the Canadian Rockies. I had skied for the very first time at age 27 on some hills in Cincinnati, Ohio. Sean was an excellent skier as he grew up in Ontario, Canada, and lived in Germany during his high school years. We had previously skied together in Maine, Colorado and West Virginia.

Skiing in Banff, Alberta, amped up my stress levels. It zapped all my energy to ski, which requires a big hunk of coordination and balance, not to mention strength. This also ate every ounce of patience I had by accentuating my deficiencies—both real and imagined. On this trip together, I was not a pleasant person. I was biting Sean's head off in direct correlation to how insecure I felt in my own body. I felt terrible for my behavior toward him that weekend, but the emotions looming inside of me just surged out. He had a purpose for our little side trip. He proposed to me in a lovely little tapas restaurant in Banff. I can only imagine what was going through his mind about what he was signing up for.

We were seated next to a beautiful piece of artwork that was painted by a local artist. We talked with the owner and we both decided to buy it and take home a piece of our history together. Like most couples, we had our fair share of not seeing things eye to eye. But we were both committed to each other and that would be enough, I thought. That next fall Sean and I were married in a small ceremony at Orton Plantation, south of Wilmington, with the specific intention of starting our own family. Sean and I were practical and realistic, considering adoption as well as conceiving biologically depending on how my cards had been dealt genetically. I had been aware that I had a 50 percent chance of showing symptoms of hereditary Ataxia in my lifetime since I was nine. We got a keg of our favorite beer, Carlsberg, a Danish pilsner to be tapped at our wedding reception, which was held at the beach house that my dad and all three of my brothers rented. Peggy joined them, as she and my dad had been partners for six years already. They all flew down from Indiana to Wilmington, North Carolina, together. Scott and Todd were similarly unstable despite their eight-year age difference and similar age of Ataxia onset. Scott's rate of progression appeared to have already caught up to Todd's. Brian had recently been tested and was negative.

After we got married, I went to have my blood drawn to be sent off to Athena Diagnostics which would definitively tell me if I had been born with or without this mutation. Athena recommended that I come back to the clinic when my results came back so a genetic counselor could deliver my results to me face to face. I quickly said,

"Oh no, I need to know my results over the phone and *immediately* when they are received." I had spent my entire life wondering "what if," and when the results came back, I needed to know right then. So it was around noon on December 28, 2006, and I was at work at UNC-Chapel Hill when the genetic counselor called me to tell me I had tested positive for Spinocerebellar Ataxia-Type 2 (SCA2).

I remember going into the bathroom and looking in the mirror, sobbing for the person who was looking back at me. It was a new position and my M.O. "appear as if everything is fine" was in full force. But this reality was overwhelming, so I just left unannounced. I still had a few hours to myself before I needed to pick up Sean from his 12-hour day shift at the hospital. I got there early, and minutes felt like hours as I waited for him to come to the car and tell him I had confirmation that I tested positive for SCA2. I remember we both cried, but then there is not much more that I recall after that. I was busy planning for the next phase of my life. I didn't have time to sit back and never contemplated not cultivating the seeds I had already planted.

HEADS OR TAILS

I was constantly around babies and young children at family gatherings on my dad's side and loved to interact with them. As a teenager, my mother had told me that I would not be able to have children, but I still aspired to have a family. I was angry at my mom for telling me what I was going to do about something that I valued probably as much as anything. I didn't tell her that I was, I just knew I would figure out a way to do it. I knew far less about Ataxia as a teenager than I know now. From what little I knew I was 100 percent sure that I could not bring a life into this world knowing they would suffer from the condition. And the age of onset was all over the board, as early as 12 in my cousin Mike and as early as two in the literature. None of my older brothers had children, and if I didn't pass this on to the next generation, SCA2 in my immediate family would end with me.

Chapter III. Wrestle with Despair

My practically set-in-stone conviction did not leave much wiggle room for Sean. His being supportive of me was not in question. However, he had his own life experience, which did not include knowing how and why I felt so strongly about this. He was about to find out. Within three weeks of our wedding, I was pregnant. Excitement was coupled with fear as I knew that I had to get tested. In the back of my mind, I had already resigned myself to thinking I must always prepare for the day I would find out that I had it. But I had never contemplated being pregnant when I found out. It was December 2006—I was now working at the Carolina Population Center at UNC in a new position. These events are outlined from documentation I kept from my medical record.

Duke University Medical Center,
Genetics New Patient Evaluation

12/12/06—Patient is 5 weeks pregnant. She requests DNA testing to determine status in patient (Dana) of trinucleotide repeat disorder, SCA2. Results expected in two to three weeks, will contact her by phone. If she is positive, she will do prenatal testing to determine status of fetus.

12/28/06—patient positive result for SCA2, phoned to patient by GC. Patient is 7 weeks pregnant.

I had just been informed that I did in fact have this condition. My mind immediately attached itself to the idea that now my passing this condition on would only be a 50 percent chance. I scheduled a chorionic villus sampling (CVS) test, where a needle would take a sample of the placental tissue to determine the status of the fetus. This technique cannot be used until 10 to 12 weeks of pregnancy. So we waited until January when I had the CVS procedure. My convictions were about to be put to the test, and although Sean supported my decision, he must have had his own convictions that he kept to himself.

On January 12, 2007, we found out the fetus tested positive for SCA2. Finding this out was gut-wrenching—I would have this pregnancy terminated. I would be the one to determine my fate—and the road that was being paved to go down could have been exactly how my mom's fateful demise started, but I would not go down this one. I was so afraid of giving into powerful emotions associated with knowing that the condition that ravaged my mom was now at work within me. I was deep in the rabbit hole of despair, as pregnancy allowed me to feel as human as I ever wanted to feel, but just as quickly reminded me that my path might never be like I had envisioned. I reacted with clockwork action. Within weeks of agonizing through this loss, I was devising a new plan.

Ongoing Injury

After going through the termination of my pregnancy, I did not want to ever go through another one again. I learned about Preimplantation Genetic Diagnosis (PGD) testing and how it can screen fertilized embryos and determine, prior to implantation into the uterus, which embryos are affected with Ataxia and which are not. Only *unaffected embryos* would be implanted. This process requires the patient to undergo the full IVF protocol, as the body is prepped to simulate a pregnancy prior to implantation that will hopefully lead to a pregnancy.

Multiple fertility centers were near Durham, but when Sean and I met with one of the doctors, he seemed overly sterile and detached. We picked Dr. Young at a clinic outside of the Triangle area. We chose him specifically because he had experience utilizing PGD and did research as well. Sean and I attended an educational session with an educator about how IVF and PGD work. Soon after, I researched several options and I picked Genesis Genetics in Detroit to develop a test specific to SCA2. DNA swabs of Sean, myself, affected brother Scott, unaffected brother Brian and my father were all used. I talked with Dr. Mark Hughes, the director at Genesis Genetics, at length about the entire process.

Sean gave me regular IVF shots and then finally it was egg retrieval day. Twelve of our fertilized embryos had survived long enough and biopsied cells were sent to Genesis Genetics in Detroit.

They would do the PGD testing to determine which embryos were affected. PGD testing was performed based on the specific test that Genesis developed over the course of weeks. Of the 12 total embryos tested, *five were unaffected,* seven were affected. On a subsequent call the clinic asked me if the seven affected embryos could be used for medical research instead of being discarded. I, of course, agreed that they could keep the affected embryos for research purposes. On September 28, 2007, Dr. McDonald performed the transfer procedure, assisted by Jim the embryologist, whom I had spoken to over the phone several times. Our doctor Dr. Young was not available that day.

I was pregnant for the second time, this time using PGD which also requires IVF, to ensure that SCA2 would not be passed to the next generation. We believed that there was little to no chance that this embryo had SCA2, so our fears disappeared, and we happily indulged in the dream of our future child. We felt confident in the PGD results done in Detroit and that the doctor had implanted one of the five unaffected embryos. We had ultrasounds in October, toured the birth center in Chapel Hill in preparation for our upcoming prenatal treatment and delivery. In early December, we told our family and friends. We prepared to become parents.

In late November, again I underwent CVS testing of the baby. When I told one of the nurses at the fertility clinic that I was having this done she replied, "You know you don't need to do that, right?" I knew the likelihood was incredibly small, but it was possible that the lab in Detroit could have encountered errors when they tested the biopsies of the embryos. I was not interested in taking any chances. While awaiting the results, Sean and I listened to the baby's heartbeat on several occasions. Our mindset for almost three months— a child was on the way that would break this cycle once and for all.

On Tuesday, December 17, 2007, at 4:00 p.m., Sydney, the genetic counselor from prenatal medicine, called. "I do not have good news. The baby tested positive for SCA2. I know there is a 1 to 2 percent chance of this—I'm sorry." At 4:20, I called the clinic and left a message for both Marsha, the IVF nurse, and Dr. Young, informing him directly that I just got the results of the CVS testing. The baby tested positive for SCA2 at 15 weeks. I kept a notebook and documented everything that happened. At the time, I couldn't tell you why I did this—I was just compelled to write everything down. *If it's not documented, it didn't happen.* I wrote these words.

complete devastation
anger
hopelessness
disbelief

Deep in my gut, I knew that it was more than chance that placed us in this situation. I had talked at length with the lab in Detroit and specifically with Dr. Mark Hughes, the director. He explained how they were going to create their test and I was impressed by multiple levels of safeguards they were using. I knew it was more likely that an error had been made by a human. I wrote out the possible errors in my notebook. On Wednesday, December 18, Dr. Young called. "I know the CVS test is right, the baby tested positive for SCA2. We made a terrible mistake." I got little to no sleep that night, my heart pounding, anxious.

On Wednesday, December 18, I had a pre-op visit for termination of the pregnancy. I slept on and off until 3 a.m. Sean could not sleep, and he had gone out to the couch. He was sobbing— I laid there with him the rest of the night. On Thursday, December 19, embryologist Jim (9:50 a.m.) and Dr. Young (5 p.m.) called me and said "they were sorry." Jim, the embryologist, and Dr. McDonald, who was scheduled to do my implantation, had mistakenly transferred one of the seven embryos affected with SCA2 instead of one of the five unaffected embryos. They blamed their failure to properly file the PGD test results from the lab in Detroit.

They had treated me with the same care and safeguards that they used with the other 98 percent of the population who walked in their door to have this implantation procedure done for IVF without PGD. It didn't matter if they misfiled my results in the cafeteria. Neither Dr. McDonald nor Jim were aware that I was there that day as a PGD patient. They were in the business of maximizing my chance of getting pregnant, except I was there for PGD in addition to IVF. I was in the 2 percent of the population and it was screaming in my face every day that I was different. Surely, they *should* know this, but I looked like everyone else who showed up for IVF—"choose the best looking, healthy embryo" is the name of the game.

A complex medical procedure that hinged on utilizing all the subsequent steps in two institutions from across the country and a handful of human beings, three of whom that day made the choice to assume that the other two would handle the details. The ten months it took to choose a clinic, undergo the IVF protocol, retrieve my eggs, fertilize with Sean's sperm, take and send biopsies from the embryos that survived, develop the test to perform the genetic test, test all twelve embryos proved to be futile since the embryologist decided that the healthiest-looking embryo was one of the seven affected with SCA2.

Thursday, December 19, 2007, was the scheduled pregnancy termination. I reached out to and talked to Liza, my best friend from childhood. Friday brought the same feelings as Thursday. I had tried to get out in the afternoon but came home and was nauseous. I reached out and talked to Sofia, my good friend from college, and then took two Percocet to sleep. It was almost Christmas, but I was not up for being with family or friends—anyone who knew what had just happened but surely didn't understand or hurt like we were hurting.

The seeds of fear had taken root in Sean now, as he also felt the very real and devastating effects of this disease. He had lived through his own loss twice now. A loss others just didn't quite understand. During a personal crisis it can feel almost impossible to step back and think about others. During this time, my own suffering was magnified, and it was too difficult to wrap my mind around the fact that Sean was suffering simultaneously and very differently than I was. I realize that the pregnancy termination procedure we had been through is experienced by many people in all kinds of circumstances all the time. And it is often gone through silently, without kind words and compassionate actions like so many other forms of loss will bring.

I called several malpractice law firms in North Carolina, none of whom appeared to comprehend what had happened. When I called an attorney referral service I was told they "cannot help me" as there was no "ongoing injury." I would beg to differ. Someone just *has to* understand. I looked online and I found out that Nancy Hersh in San Francisco had represented a woman who was a victim of embryo mix-up, which was as close as I could get to what had just happened to us. I immediately called her. As soon as I explained our situation to her and what happened, she immediately agreed to take the case—she got it. Months later, she flew to North Carolina and we met with her prior to the mediation that was scheduled.

This loss was magnified far beyond the technical error that was so obvious. This was also directly due to multiple human beings who were able to overlook the sole purpose for our presence in their clinic. Had Dr. Young been present that day, I am ninety-nine percent sure this mistake would not have been made. The face to face meetings Sean and I had with him forced a connection that was nowhere to be found with Dr. McDonald, whom I had never met until the day of the transfer. I know it was not rational, but I could not help but feel as if this mistake was directly related to my Ataxia. It was in fact the opposite—because no one could visibly detect my slight symptoms, they lumped me into the majority of IVF patients. Dr. Young was intimately familiar with our story, but he was not there. "The matter was resolved," but that was little compensation for the devastation they had unknowingly perpetuated.

A Child's Hope

After I was diagnosed in 2006, I got a new neurologist. It would be like Christmas and I would see him once a year for a lifetime. The very first gift Dr. Burton Scott gave me was a piece of paper with National Ataxia Foundation (NAF) written on it. I would frequent the NAF webpage (ataxia.org) as I wanted to learn as much as I could and find out about who was doing research and where and when events were being held. I would also learn, and it was initially uncomfortable to read the details of how I would begin to lose my fine motor skills and balance until eventually swallowing and breathing would become impossible due to the degeneration of the cerebellum, which is the part of the brain located at the base of the skull and provides coordination, balance, and vital functions like swallowing and breathing.

The more I read, the more comfortable I became with that knowledge because the more I thought about it, I was one of the lucky ones that wasn't symptomatic in my teens or 20s like my cousins were. I was diagnosed at age 34 and was not clinically symptomatic until almost 40. My first cousins were diagnosed in their teens and were lucky to live until 34. The atrocities that Ataxia had already doled out to members of my family were far worse than what I was dealing with. My education in exercise physiology and my career in research had allowed me to silently wonder and hypothesize my own questions for the next 10 years.

One thing I didn't hypothesize about was whether I could bring a child into this world knowing the risk of passing this on to them. I had made the decision as a teen that this was not going to happen and the only way that I was going to have a baby biologically was if I was sure I did not carry the mutation. Because of my mother point blank telling me I could not have children, I had contemplated adoption since then. I had a good childhood friend who was adopted, and I didn't see her life as being any different than mine or any of my other friends. Not having a family of my own was not something I could fathom.

Sean was aware from soon after we met the possibility that I carried the gene that may or may not cause Ataxia. We had considered adoption as well as biological children or both. We had discussed adopting from China, where we had visited his parents in Beijing in 2004 where they were living and teaching. China had recently changed its policy requiring couples be married for three years before even applying, so we didn't consider this for long. Then we had considered adopting from Guatemala, until its relations with the United States became strained and adoptions between the countries came to a halt.

In early 2008, Sean and I made the decision to go forward to officially get placed on a local adoption agency's waiting list. We met with a social worker from the agency to resume the process we had started months earlier. We attended the required meetings and were assigned a social worker to help us navigate all the paperwork. It took several weeks but I steamrolled through the long list of requirements. We were so fortunate to be matched with a birth mom by late July 2008. From the time we were matched to "Birth mom X" late in her pregnancy to the day she gave birth was only seven days. Kendall came home with us when she was eight days old.

The moment we received a call from our social worker telling us we had been matched with a birth mother my maternal instincts kicked into high gear. This was what I had been yearning for my entire life—being a mom. Kendall gave me a sense of purpose as well as a 24/7 reminder of the power that unconditional love can bring. I had just been placed working at the Duke Center for Health Policy Research by a contract agency without a contingency for maternal leave from work. In July 2008 when I was placed there, I would have never dreamed that we would adopt a baby within my first 30 days there. The center graciously gave me my requested two weeks off to be home and bond with Kendall and then I gradually started back part- and then full-time within a month. Sean would take a break from working full-time and would stay home with her while I was at work on weekdays.

This was a far cry from how I envisioned this scenario would go. Up until that point, Sean and I agreed that I would be the primary stay-at-home parent for our child. But Sean was becoming increasingly drained, working the night shift in the burn center. It made sense that I stay in my new position given that I had just been placed at Duke. I still wasn't clinically symptomatic at this time, but I wanted to start immersing myself and my family in doing something, anything but nothing. Staying in my position while Sean stayed home seemed to have worked out for the best as I was hired into a permanent position at Duke by the end of the year. And if I needed to, I would bring Kendall to the office with me, still in her infant seat.

I had already scoured the National Ataxia Foundation website (ataxia.org) for information. Baltimore was hosting an annual picnic for families with Ataxia and it was a five-hour drive from Durham. When Kendall was 13 months old, Sean drove us up to Baltimore, Maryland, to Johns Hopkins University Ataxia Center. This would be my first experience with a National Ataxia Foundation event. We listened to professional and non-professional speakers, had lunch and talked with several other families. After the official program was complete, I noticed a man working with individuals. He was having some of them walk back and forth and others were walking up and down stairs. After watching for a while, I managed to get a word with him. He was a former surgeon who also had Ataxia, Dr. Tom Clouse. He was talking to others about how they could focus their energy on certain aspects of walking and balance that could be helpful to remain mobile and utilize their assets for as long as possible.

I was interested in learning more about what he did. We emailed back and forth in 2009 and luckily Dr. Clouse had a son who lived in Raleigh and he had already planned a trip here. I discussed this with my brother, Scott, and he agreed to fly down from Indiana to our house to meet with him. Tom arrived at our house in Durham in his travel camper. He talked with both of us, but Tom gravitated to help Scott with his walking as he was noticeably further advanced than me. Scott walked on flat surfaces, up and down stairs and he got up and down from a seated position. After an hour or so Scott was not incredibly receptive to what he was suggesting—work against what your body is telling you and make a conscious effort to resist what comes naturally. I was more than receptive to his ideas and they took root in my mind. Below is from his website in 2017.

Key Concepts to Understand

Throughout this process of re-learning how to walk and move I found some obvious problems I had to change. My movements had become anything but normal, and you are doing the same thing. Gradually we have modified our movements to accommodate our changing neurological condition [www.walkingwithAtaxia.com].

Dr. Clouse was one of those people that I was incredibly fortunate to have crossed paths with in Baltimore. I immediately "got" what he was saying and think I even subconsciously tucked away his theories about how to envision moving until I would need them. Ten years later, when I walk, I am continually thinking about "lifting my knee to move my foot," not just lifting my foot to walk.

Jamie Heywood is another example of someone I feel fortunate to have crossed paths with, but in a much more random way. While I was working for the Center for Personalized Medicine at Duke in 2012, I attended a talk given by Jamie, who was on campus from Boston. As with many health-related presentations, the title can be misleading. This one was titled something like "Patient Recruitment" so I walked across campus to the Duke Clinical Research Institute (DCRI) to hear his presentation, not knowing who he was. I was a clinical research coordinator and I had learned the importance of getting the patient's perspective in order to maximize participation rates.

My expectations could not have been more off base as he started his presentation with a tribute to his younger brother who had suffered from and died of ALS, or Lou Gehrig's disease. Jamie explained how he had developed a web-based patient tool where the patient enters their own health data. It was designed for patients afflicted with any condition to go and find meaningful data that relates to their condition. Often patients are given clinical data, without any guidance on how this information affects their everyday life. I spoke briefly with Jamie after the talk and went home and created an account and started entering my data on www.patientslikeme.com. I entered my data so it could potentially help someone else easily access what has been helpful to me.

I entered my data in hopes it might potentially help someone else, but I was also going through the process of identifying what information was relevant to me. Most advances in clinical care are the result of an analysis of a clinical trial. When you participate in a clinical trial you also agree to allow researchers to use your data the way they want to use it. Clinical data can be used clinically and for research, but research data can only be used for research. Why can't research data be used to inform our choices clinically? Why can't research studies include some predetermined basic clinical measures that can be released to a treating physician, if requested? For a neurology patient who typically has only one visit a year, more measures could add insight to clinical care.

Chapter IV

A Complex Machine

The brain is a complex biological organ possessing immense computational capability: it constructs our sensory experience, regulates our thoughts and emotions, and controls our actions.—Eric Kandel

There's No I in Team

Although my 15-year stint on the court was long over, the basketball mindset stayed with me. I excelled in the environment of a team. Everyone was working toward the same goal. It was exhilarating to take the cues provided by the coach and help set them in motion out on the court. Although I felt mostly disconnected from my basketball career, I continued to have a strong passion for fighting for what I wanted. Despite having worked for both universities and living smack-dab between UNC and Duke, I'm not a huge fan of either one. I am usually behind their opponent, rooting for the underdog.

What I learned through basketball was that maintaining your role on a team of any kind is fraught with unexpected hardships. Basketball gave me a chance to adapt to an ever-changing role based on circumstances. Your relative position to the ball was constantly changing. One of my favorite things to do was help defend against an unsuspecting opponent who knew they had beaten a teammate of mine. I could shift over and provide last-second help-side defense. From elementary through high school, I flowed between floundering newbie to poised leader. In college, I fulfilled these same roles, but my offensive prowess was overshadowed by the majority on my team.

There was still a need for a workhorse who was thrilled to go in for defensive purposes and happily filled the role of a consistent and hard-working sub. My coach, Bill Fennelly, had recruited me to Toledo. He was an animated, fiery sergeant with a hair trigger. If a teammate got cussed out by him during practice, we would all give her our support and encouragement. In games, if anyone was playing outside of their role or being selfish, someone would step up and tell them to get their act together. We were constantly keeping each other in line and had each other's back.

Sean knew very early into our relationship the risk that I had of having Ataxia. His acknowledgment and acceptance were reassuring and yet purely abstract at that point. We had been together for five years and had lived together before we got married, so marriage was a technicality for us before we started a family. However, after the romance of our small beach wedding and celebration, life wasn't exactly as smooth sailing as the previous five years had been. My diagnosis just weeks after tying the knot threw a permanent crease in my slacks. After my diagnosis, I had this fierce determination inside me that said "ain't nothing going to drag me down!" Unknowingly, this began as my intention to "do something" which morphed into "do anything." We were only two years into our marriage in 2008, and Sean and I had suffered more hardships during this time than we could have ever imagined.

Unlike this flow that I was so used to, the hardships Sean and I experienced drove a wedge between us so deep that utilizing our own coping mechanisms camouflaged each other's wounds and needs. Sean and I were no longer on the same team fighting the same battle. We had formed our own teams in order to survive. My wheels were constantly spinning about how we could work through our differences—books, counseling, talking it through. I was always coming up with a new game plan, and I felt Sean was always glued to the bench.

In October 2008, I emailed Sean.

_____

Sean,

I feel very disconnected to you and this makes me sad. I'm sorry if I seem too demanding, but I'm truly only seeking happiness and togetherness. I cannot seem to say the right words to express this and I feel like my requests are being construed into nagging. I really don't know what to do and feel very alone in the struggle as when I bring anything up to you, things are "fine." I don't even know what I'm asking of you and feel somewhat desperate that I am emailing this because I feel speaking with you only aggravates things. We need to come up with a solution that we are both comfortable with and my ears are open.

Love, D

Sean may or may not have responded, I don't recall. But his inaction to my ongoing plea made me feel helpless, like I had never stated my desires. When I told Sean what I wanted and where I wanted us to be, I felt like he would never acknowledge what I had said. Effectively, I had spoken but I had felt like I had not been heard. There were multiple options to fix the problem, and I was convinced that I just hadn't found the right one yet. As complications surfaced throughout the first years of our marriage, I became more skeptical that we would someday overcome the mounting distance that was building between us.

FUEL TO THE FIRE

Already navigating my marriage to Sean in a leaky boat, my brother Scott's suicide on February 28, 2011, was like a jagged rock that ripped a gaping hole in it. His suicide was his escape route from what was in his mind a no-win situation with Ataxia. My dad, who had already been deeply traumatized 18 years earlier after finding his wife's body, had also found his youngest son's. This had been planned and carefully thought through, just like my mom had done. Scott had lived in a house with Todd just down the road from my dad's cabin. He had driven his car to my dad's secluded cabin in the wooded hills of Brown County. When Dad returned home from visiting us in Durham, he found Scott in his driveway. There would be no one home. Scott shot himself in the head.

Sean and I were both knocked off our feet with shock. My grief was intense, and it seeped out steadily and uncontrollably. My eyes stayed puffy and red for days. Sean tried to console me. My feeling was that a part of me had died too. The part of me that was tethered to Scott by our sibling status and shared illness. The part of me that had tried to bring him over to the other side, the side where he would not keep suffering more and more until there was no return. My grief was a horrifying reminder that like my mom's life, Scott's life could not be recreated or imagined by anyone else. And they both chose to put an end to theirs.

In a surprising and confusing phone call, my dad insisted that we not make a trip back to Indiana. We would have a memorial service back in Warsaw this coming summer. This coming summer? I was angry at Scott for doing this at our dad's house and angry at my dad that we would not get to grieve our loss together. This felt so wrong, but I also felt I needed to respect my dad's wishes. It felt wrong because not coming home also meant that I couldn't acknowledge my own grief to the remaining members of my dwindling family.

While I was writing about Scott, I called Peter Davis, one of his best friends from Ball State in Muncie, Indiana. He said that his freshman year Scott told him he was pretty sure he had it. He told him that he was definitely seeing symptoms by 1997, when he was 26. That year was when he left Paris and moved to Brazil where he got married in 2000.

After the relationship ended, he returned to Indiana in 2004. It was clear that he was now visibly struggling physically and emotionally with his new reality. He had been symptomatic for almost a decade but kept it a secret, honoring a family tradition. Sean, Kendall and I traveled to Warsaw that May, when our family held a memorial service that my dad led. My dad had constructed a large mural with photographs and brought Scott's ashes in an urn. My dad read from his notes as he neatly and thoroughly summarized Scott's

Opposite: **Scott Creighton near his sixth-floor apartment on this street in Paris, France, 1994.**

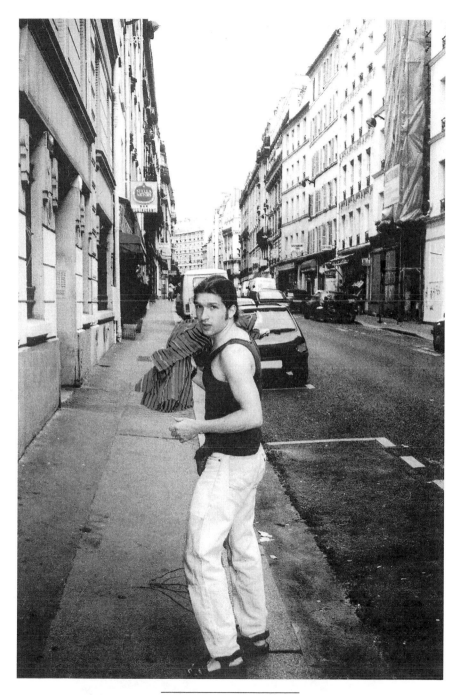

life and his spirit. Only our immediate family and close friends of Scott attended as we shared stories and memories of him. Peter, one of his closest friends, had to stop in the middle and compose himself as he played guitar and sang "Bob Dylan's Dream," a favorite from within their inner circle. I sat listening while I sobbed for his soul that could never be replaced. I believe that when Scott knew he was starting to show symptoms, he did his part to live his life to its fullest in the abbreviated timeframe his abilities would allow him to. After Scott's death, I admitted that I would need and accept all the help I could get for the rest of my life.

My own version of "Bob Dylan's Dream" was unfolding in front of me. Several months after Scott's suicide, I was offered and accepted a new full-time position within the university. This was a lateral move, but a welcomed change. In my new position, I was contracted out to provide support to various health-related research projects that needed coordination across campus. During the first few weeks in my new position, I struggled to focus on the steadily increasing number of projects I was responsible for. Cheryl, my hiring supervisor, asked to meet with me prior to the 90-day probationary period that is required for all employees new to any department at Duke. I was called out for not performing up to expectations and was told I was proving unable to fulfill my assigned tasks.

I felt betrayed that this was the first and only conversation with me about my performance since I had started there. Cheryl also told me that Dr. Bingham did not want to work with me anymore. After I promptly addressed these concerns directly with Dr. Bingham, she stated that Cheryl had taken her comments out of context. This fueled my rage toward Cheryl, who was for the first time presenting herself as heartless and two-faced. What I was secretly angry about was her assumption that I was not capable. She had no idea what was adding fuel to the fire, but I was quick to judge her for her failure to see what was so obvious to me.

For the first time in my life, at 38, I felt like my world was unraveling both personally and professionally and I had little control to manipulate the outcome. Kendall, now three, had frequent night terrors. She would fall asleep then wake up crying and screaming. Sean was starting back at UNC on the night shift, so I would take Kendall into bed with me in the other bedroom so he could get a full night's sleep. I was already waking a lot each night in anticipation of the next workday and now I was soothing Kendall back to sleep before I could go back to sleep too. Sleep deprivation on top of feeling overwhelmed in a new job seemed like a recipe for disaster.

Each doctor I worked with had different dispositions and had a need for my work to fulfill a portion of their currently funded project. Each project required a different aspect of coordination—making copies, writing standard operating procedures, completing regulatory forms, and interacting directly with patients. Performing each task individually was not a concern; it was constantly shifting gears and performing each one separately that proved difficult. All required a different level of fine motor skills and mine were slowly diminishing which added to the stress, rapidly elevating my symptoms. The anticipation of what task was coming next while trying to focus on the current one was overwhelming and exhausting physically and mentally.

Each doctor independently communicated clearly with me, and over time it was apparent to me that I was falling short of expectations. This incrementally dialed up my stress level and made each workday more challenging. I can remember walking across campus to the Sickle Cell office building. Cheryl had already disclosed my difficulties to Dr. Bingham. I was rushing to get there on time, having just made copies of forms for the patients and the entire Sickle Cell team. I remember as I got closer and closer my legs got heavier and heavier, as if my feet were covered in concrete.

During this time, I was in frequent contact with my department human resources office. They made me aware of all of my options. I also had a visit with my PCP, who gave me a short supply of anti-anxiety meds to help me get through the workday and to sleep. I wouldn't rely on them for long, as I decided that I would leave this position and take a short hiatus to regain my composure on Family Medical Leave of Absence (FMLA). Luckily, the project I had been working on from my previous position was going well. I was already functioning at the top of my learning curve for this project, so it was a comparative breeze to keep it going.

My former department knew the short story that it was not working out, and when they offered me my position back, I was relieved and grateful for how this situation worked out. When I returned to the Center for Personalized Medicine, they agreed to my request to only work 20 hours per week. I did this just to be safe, and with no questions asked by my old department. Then I moved back up to 30 hours per week to maintain my health benefits. "Thank God this crisis was averted just in time," I thought to myself.

March Madness

Parting ways can be recognizing that two perfectly flawed humans may be on different life paths. Not because of a conscious choice but rather following an instinctive drive. It became apparent to me that I wasn't the only one suffering symptoms of depression. Sean and I discussed it and he agreed to go see his doctor, who prescribed an antidepressant. I felt a sense of relief that some of the darkness in his background might be lifted. Looking back, I wonder if his agreement to get treatment was simply a method to shut me up. The closeness we once had seemed so distant and his touch now felt foreign and forced. And when Sean made a concerted effort toward intimacy, it became harder for me to reciprocate physically and emotionally. As I pulled away physically, he pulled back emotionally, and this cycled back and forth.

At this time, I wasn't familiar with the five languages of love. I would later read and discover that my need for close connection and physical touch that I had relied on for my entire life was now drifting further and further away. I knew I would have a reliable connection with my best friend, Julie. I drove up to Danville, Virginia, to visit her overnight. She was probably eight months pregnant with her daughter. We were talking after dinner when I received a mistaken text from Sean. He accidentally texted me instead of his friend Mark that he would be by soon with a six-pack. This is not an incident that I would find alarming, except he had purposely not disclosed these plans to me. I was furious at him and at the state of our marriage and I certainly didn't disguise this from Julie. This was one example of why I was feeling that the trust we once had might be harder to find than I had thought.

Months had passed since my brother Scott's death. As Sean and I were bickering about something trivial I said something about his antidepressant. He responded, "I stopped taking those months ago." My blood began to boil as I thought back over the last several months and how I was giving him repeated benefits of the doubt that he was doing his best. But he had taken the initiative to stop his medication and not considered it important that he inform me. Withholding information from me was a stark reminder from my past that not knowing the truth felt a lot worse than knowing. It was, to me, a conscious betrayal of our trust.

My professional career had effectively brainwashed my mind to focus on the positive—striving to always improve, for better wellness, health prevention and interventions that may be helpful. It was now 2012, six years into our marriage and after my diagnosis. What I had been preparing myself for most of my life was in full effect, no more dress rehearsals. Sean was trying to figure out how to take our reality as a family forward into the future. He was always looking past the present moment, as if he could make future plans without having to attach feelings related to my health.

Yet how could he plan our future while trying to forget about what happened to my mom and now my brother? He would always shift our conversations to the future, trips to take, places to go. I was convinced that by not allowing himself to engage in the present, we would never share any enjoyment in the future. His goals were looking ahead to tomorrow, next week, next month, and my goals were finding happiness together, today. Our continually diverging roads were leading us in different directions with certainly separate destinations.

Sean's parents lived in Ontario, Canada, and were spending the winter months down at the beach in North Carolina. They had not seen Kendall in a while, and they invited us down for a visit. Sean decided to stay home to pick up a night shift at the hospital that weekend. This was the first time Kendall and I would go down to visit his parents without him. I felt that our trust was nonexistent and as if our marriage was hanging together by threads. I had even been in the habit of very purposely, as a signal to him, verbalizing my discontent. Was it also a conscious admission to myself that I was letting go of reconciliation?

I had recently gotten a rash on my ring finger, which was rather peculiar, like wearing it actually felt toxic. I conveniently used this as the reason to take off my ring. It was white gold with a blue sapphire surrounded by small diamonds. Sean offered to take it to the jeweler to get it cleaned while I was away for the weekend. Prior to going to the beach without Sean, I was already frantically looking for an escape from our commitment. I came up with nothing substantial or concrete, other than the fact that I felt alone in my journey to a more fulfilling life. In my mind, that wasn't going to be nearly enough. But if you look for something hard enough, you are likely to find it.

It was in the middle of March Madness and Sean's Canadian parents did not share in my excitement for this magical time. They did not have cable in their part-time beach townhome either. Friday night when Kendall and I arrived, we had dinner at their house. Then I went to the nearby country club so I could watch the live games. When I entered by myself, there were big screen TVs with the games going on, but since dinner was being served, the sound was turned off. Watching the games with no sound was slightly torturous for me. The next day, we all spent the day taking Kendall to the beach and shopping in nearby Southport, a quaint little coastal town nearby.

By Saturday evening, I was amazed at how energized I felt. I was already in my happy place, as the NCAA Tournament is the most wonderful time of the year. I love to witness the tooth-and-nail battles that often lead to stunning upsets. I was reeling from intensely happy feelings after spending the day at the beach with Kendall. I decided to go somewhere different to watch the games Saturday night, with sound this time. I still had on my beach clothes, flip flops and ballcap. And since it was tournament time, I also had on my game face. I sat down at the sports bar in the only open seat, down at the far end. From the corner of my eye, I spotted an older man and was relieved by the fact that he had a full head of gray hair; this was "safe."

I exchanged hellos with the two men who were seated next to me and we introduced ourselves. Barry, sitting to my left, and I had an immediate but unspecified connection. I was drawn to his tanned and handsome face, blue eyes and striking head of silver hair. He was there with his friend Max. When Barry asked why I was on the island I threw my cards on the table. I blurted out that I was here visiting my in-laws for the weekend with my three-year-old daughter.

Ohio State was playing Cincinnati in the "Elite Eight" of the NCAA Tournament in March 2012. The three of us all had ties to Ohio. I played basketball at the University of Toledo, Barry grew up in Ohio and Max graduated from a university in Ohio.

Barry appeared to be at least 10 years older than me and Max may have been 10 years younger. The three of us continued talking throughout the first game and we watched as Ohio State defeated Cincinnati. When the game was over, they got up to leave and we said goodbye. As they walked out, I felt a little pang of "damn." But then Barry came back to ask me if I wanted to meet somewhere else for a drink, as he was going to run Max back to the house. I said "absolutely" as I was happy to continue our "conversation."

When it was the three of us, we talked about basketball or Ohio. Now, we were free to take it anywhere. We talked about food, music, growing up in the Midwest, and church. Barry was active with a local church on the island. I told him that when Kendall was an infant, we started going to a non-denominational church in Durham. Nothing shared was incredibly personal, and it was just an easy conversation. I do remember that once we realized that it was getting late, things tensed up a bit as neither one of us wanted to part ways yet.

When he asked me if I wanted to come to his place, it did not hold a sexual connotation for me. It seemed innocuous—his friend was there, and it was on my way home as well. And I had already put my cards on the table when we had first met: "I am here visiting my in-laws."

On the way out, as we walked to our cars, I could feel my own imbalance, after a few beers. Rather than wondering if he noticed it too, I volunteered that I had a balance disorder, and that was why my walking was unsteady. We arrived at the house after midnight and Max had already gone to bed. We continued talking on the screened in porch, facing each other in chairs. I have no recollection of what we were talking about but we both leaned forward and began to kiss. We both were on the same page now, so we hurried upstairs to the bedroom. We were tearing our clothes off and we made love with a passion that I didn't even know was possible.

My mind was completely blind to the implications of what I was doing. I was so completely in that moment, enjoying our emotional connection that had been building all night and the physical connection we had just shared. The connection that started in our minds and then our bodies. Let's just say that we were both apparently in need of the same thing. We were two vulnerable human beings who stripped off more than our clothes. I will only speak for myself in saying that I found exactly what I had been searching for. I had found a meaningful connection with someone who acknowledged what I had said and accepted me as I was. Even if it was only for a few hours, it was now a bona fide reality and not just a crazy pipe-dream.

TRANSFORMATION

I was completely in the moment and had totally given over to this spontaneous experience. When the pleasure ended, not only my consciousness but maybe my conscience caught up with the rest of me. We were both staring up at the ceiling when I said out loud to myself and to Barry, "I'm still married." I believe that he was completely blindsided by this declaration. My actions that night were as authentic as I have ever been and his interpretation of my behavior all evening signaled to him that I was available. Through sex, I got something that I was craving—a meaningful connection. That intense connection paired with my perception of his absolute acceptance of me.

The next day, Barry and I took a walk on the beach. He point-blank asked me why I had not disclosed to him that I was married. I told him my whole story, that within just two months of our marriage I was diagnosed with a progressive neurologic condition. I was diagnosed by a DNA test, so the diagnosis was not even related to measurable symptoms. Five years later, I was living with minimal limitations. In my mind, I felt incredibly lucky to have a family, friends, a job, a seemingly great life. Inside, I was yearning for something with more meaning and for someone who could see me just as I was and not as I used to be. Barry never took my side or told me it was OK to feel the way I did. He posed this to me instead—maybe Sean was not capable of what I was expecting of him.

For the first time, I felt relief that what he had just said may be true, that it was not my fault for expecting what I felt I deserved nor was it Sean's fault he could not deliver what I needed. It was a relief to say this out loud to Barry, who listened and heard me. I knew from that moment on that I could no longer go back to the way things were. Verbalizing to him what I ultimately wanted allowed me to envision something different. I had finally reached my point of no return in how I thought about my life. I learned that it was all right to want more than what I was getting. In 2018, I was reading *Broken Open* by Elizabeth Lesser and felt a sense of connection to her words. She describes how reading someone else's words impacted her.

> It would take years for me to integrate what I read into my life. But at least now I understood the roots of my inability to make big and powerful decisions at home or work. I had been asking only one organ my poor brain to carry the full weight of my life. It was time to give some of the work over to my heart [38].

The day I met Barry, I was allowing my heart and spirit to guide my decisions, not just my brain, like I had learned to do my whole life. On any given day prior to then, I would have relied 99 percent on my brain to *not* make any decisions that might have led to the breakup of my marriage. I had not consciously made a connection between my act of diving in headfirst with my heart and the resulting ripples that would be created as a result, ripples that would be completely catastrophic to life as I knew it. But when I read Elizabeth Lesser's own words about her life, six years after these events happened in mine, it made sense to me in a way that gave me both relief and solace.

When I went to the beach that weekend, I had already begun to transform. I had already admitted to myself that working full-time in a new position was more than I could handle. After a short FMLA leave at work and returning to my old job at a reduced schedule, I had re-evaluated what was important to me and how I was going to live the rest of my life. Unfortunately, that meant a life without Sean as my husband. Looking back now it was a perfect storm of events that all lined up so that there was only one possible option: to leave Sean. Leaving for the beach I had been in a place of high anxiety and felt a desperation and fear that I had not felt before. Deep inside me I felt I had no choice but to make a change in my life. Although I did not realize it yet, I had already mentally prepared to go forward with a life that was meaningful and fulfilling. It was painful for us both but ultimately has led to what I believe to be a much more authentic existence for both of us.

After my return from the beach and my declaration that we would be separating in order to divorce, Sean and I agreed to cohabitate until we figured out the next step. I quickly found out this was easier said than done. I never confessed to Sean what had happened with another man that weekend. I didn't want my actions with Barry to shape Sean's perception as it being the root cause for my sudden and swift decision. Sean had mastered denying that a problem existed throughout our marriage. Now, suddenly, his feelings that he had been robbed were pouring out of him on a daily basis.

Both of us had such strong emotional reactions to what was happening that neither one of us could channel anything other than what could only be detrimental to Kendall. This was the sole home she had ever known. We both agreed Kendall should remain in the house with one of us. The lesser of two evils won and I decided I could not live this way anymore. I found an apartment nearby. I was settling in my apartment and realized my wedding ring was back at the house. I asked Sean if he had seen it and he replied "no." Red flags were waving wildly right in front of my face. My gut instinct was tripped as I knew that I had not taken it with me and I hadn't even worn it for more than a month. His claim that he "hadn't seen it" was a sure sign that he knew exactly where it was. Since we were splitting time with Kendall, I knew his work schedule.

When I knew he was not home I made a visit to see for myself. I was no longer going to ride in the back seat of my own life. Within minutes I found my ring neatly placed in a charging station that I had bought for him a few years prior. This used to sit on the bedroom furniture but now it was sitting out next to the kitchen along with his other prized possessions. Everything in the enclosed box was placed there by him. I put the ring in my pocket and checked a mark beside by name on my scorecard. I had always thought of divorce as someone else's option, not mine. Four years after our separation I wrote this but never sent it. I never would have had these insights as they were happening in real time.

Sean,

Please forgive me for not being faithful to you and for ultimately initiating our divorce. It was not a premeditated act, yet it was an experience that transformed my life by coming to the realization that not living 100% in the present moment is like not living at all. I know it took you by surprise that I came home and had such a profound change but please understand that I had undergone a transformation about how I was going to live the rest of my life and how I wanted Kendall's exposure of me to be.

I needed to know that she would see me as strong and happy not frustrated and angry all the time. I saw in my behavior toward you exactly how my mom reacted to her diagnosis and knowing her fate pushed me to resist those actions and choose a different path.

I am proud of the parent that I am and hope that you perceive me the same after we separated. I do not regret what happened. I only know that you might think I was selfish. I'm sorry I caused you pain and I know that you never would have left me, and I admire you for that. I simply could not continue the path that we were on that was filled with anger, resentment and bitterness that traveled in both directions.

I'm sorry, Dana

I was seeing a therapist in the weeks leading up to our separation. This was just after I had returned to work after my short FMLA leave. He was an excellent therapist, a social worker Sean and I had seen years ago, shortly after we were married. He was quite familiar with the problems we had been having throughout our marriage and with my diagnosis. I called him the Monday after I returned from the beach and told him I needed to meet ASAP. I told my therapist what happened with Barry. He asked me if my marriage to Sean was contingent on whether things ended up working out with Barry. My answer was a resounding "absolutely not."

Barry and I continued to talk sporadically for several weeks, even though my lawyer advised me not to. Barry ultimately told me by email that he could not continue to communicate further with me and that was our last correspondence. I was stunned and in disbelief, but I had also uncovered parts of me that I knew I could rely on like my gut instinct that I had been neatly covering up my whole life. I had found my first stepping-stone upon which I would find another and then another that would keep me from sinking down even further. I was fortunate to have multiple people impact my life like this, in meaningful ways.

I serendipitously met Ruth in 2010, before my divorce. We had each taken our daughters to the mall playground one morning to let them play early before the older, stronger kids arrived and could bulldoze over our toddlers. Annie and Kendall, who are both African American, took to each other even faster than Ruth and I did. Following their lead, we exchanged numbers so we could get together again. Since the girls loved to play, we got together often. We quickly became soul sisters as did our children. As soon as she began talking and until this day, Kendall proclaims that Annie is her sister.

Ruth and I both had careers in research, so we shared a mutual understanding of each other's work. She worked in gastrointestinal procedures research and I was in genomics research, which couldn't have been more different. Our connection ran much deeper than our careers, and I shared with her my entire story. This bonded us to each other, and we built a lasting friendship where each of us lent support to the other when it was needed. Though I had an aversion to the practice of yoga, she had become a yoga instructor and we were in tune on a spiritual level. Ruth was also a great creator and was an expert at whipping up something delicious with only the ingredients she already had. Eventually I began to pick up her style, which forced me to rely on my instincts and included never using a measuring cup again.

My instincts also led me to my divorce. As it was not a pre-planned event, I had not made arrangements for what exactly was going to happen. Before I decided to get an apartment, I wanted to make it clear that the decision to separate had been made. Ruth still owned her house in Durham after she had gotten married the previous summer and was living in a new home. I would put Kendall to bed each night, leaving her with Sean, then drive to Ruth's mostly empty house but with a bed to sleep in. I would wake up early the next morning and come home to get Kendall up and ready for her day, take her to preschool and then go to work.

When I would get to the big empty house every night I would often read or listen to CDs that I would get from the library. I had loved Lucinda Williams since my friend Julie, back in 2001, had taken me to a concert in Raleigh, and we wedged our way right to the front of the stage. I had recently discovered Lucinda's song "Blessed" and felt a deep connection to the lyrics. The local library did not carry it, so I checked out *Little Honey* instead. I stumbled upon her song "Knowing." I would listen to it over and over each night as I lay in bed, often falling asleep to it. The lyrics were incredibly powerful and shockingly familiar to what I had just experienced with Barry that weekend at the beach. Lucinda's words dance around it, but she doesn't reveal exactly what the knowing is. That's why it is so powerful to me—Barry accepted me for exactly who I was, and he listened to what I said. He didn't respond that he would help me figure out or tell me what I should do. He showed me what I needed to see. By helping me see my situation through a different perspective, he gave me permission to see an alternative that I never allowed myself to envision.

A few months passed and I was now living back in the comfort of my home. Sean had bought a house in nearby Chapel Hill. Ruth now had another toddler of her own. We saw each other considerably less often, but we still kept in touch. On one of our brief phone calls she told me I needed to listen to "Just Breathe," which was quite a bit different from the songs I had associated with Eddie Vedder. I had been a fan of Pearl Jam since high school but since that time I had not kept up with their music. Musically and lyrically, it was certainly one of the most captivating and moving songs I had ever heard. It was only recently that I fully understood why I had felt such a deep connection to this song. I wish I could have let my mom know that the pain and devastation she felt was crippling, as I can now only begin to understand. And it didn't even matter that I understood; it was that I wanted to be there for her regardless. I was willing to share her burden, but I didn't know that's what I needed to tell her.

So Much, So Fast

After separating from Sean in 2012, I started taking tiny steps back to myself. Even though I wasn't consciously making decisions that were mindful, I was filling my bucket drop by drop. I was learning that doing things that made me happy and minimizing choices led to vast improvements to my overall outlook. I chose to drive through scenic Duke Forest as opposed to taking the crowded highway to work. I shopped for clothes almost exclusively from the clearance rack. Listening to music and talk radio and watching documentaries were how I chose to spend my spare time. Making these adjustments by paring down my life in an apartment made it seem less painful.

I chose this apartment because it was near our house, it allowed dogs, and it had a short-term lease option with a pool. Kendall loved to swim, and she became really good that summer. I knew this apartment would only be a short-term solution, so I decided not to get cable or even Internet access. Without the distractions of devices, I read books, listened to CDs and watched documentaries that I would get at the library. I finally rented and watched the documentary about the life and death of Jamie Heywood's brother, Stephen, *Too Much, Too Fast*, which I had heard about from Jamie's presentation at Duke. This chronicled how Jamie identified the issues patients face which he became well aware of as his brother Stephen battled ALS. Jamie then created a tool to break down the barriers and provide patients with what they needed—data that was relevant to them. After watching this documentary, I was in awe of the actions Jamie had taken to do something groundbreaking.

After a few months, I was back in the comfort of my home. For about a year, I had been subsisting on the love of my daughter and my girlfriends, who were providing much needed support which included comedic relief.

Then I realized that my chances of ever locating a romantic partner were low, based on where I was spending all of my time. Soon after recognizing and acknowledging this in early 2013, I met Jamel. Our connection was immediate and obvious to us both. I had been ill the previous night with a fast-moving stomach bug, so the night we met for a drink I had ginger ale while we talked for probably less than an hour. He commented that he liked my energy and that surprised and intrigued me at the same time. That was the first time I had heard that from anyone.

Jamel had qualities that spoke to me in ways that I now had a new appreciation for. He grew up in southern Virginia and I in northern

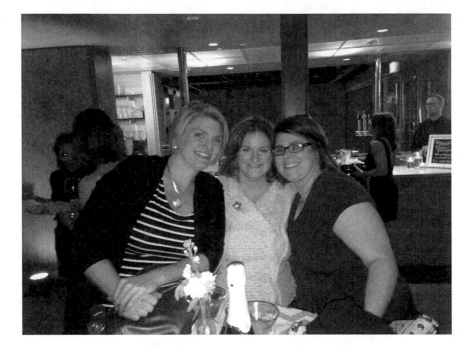

(From left) Dana Creighton, Julie Hughes and Tricia Dasilva at a friend's 40th birthday party on Franklin Street in Chapel Hill, North Carolina, 2015.

Indiana. Clearly, we had different upbringings and life experiences. Jamel utilized our differences in discussions in a way that helped me understand both how our experiences had been so drastically different and how our similarities and connection as humans ultimately outweighed those differences. His master's degree in electrical engineering was proof that his brain functioned on a different level than mine. He was named Black Engineer of the Year and he holds several patents. I still don't understand how a trained electrical engineer ends up as a near-guru in Bluetooth wireless technology, but that's another story.

The impact that Jamel had on my life was tremendous. He introduced me to a lot of music that was new to me. We used music as a form of communication, and we would send each other music that spoke to us in different ways. We spent the next several months talking, listening to music or cooking and having dinner. When we did become intimate, it was something that deepened our already solid connection. I felt a sense of great relief when I was able to release not only my thoughts and unbridled opinions but a sexual energy that reminded me of my own humanity. We were both working and were lucky to get together twice a week. When we did see each other, it was quality time. There was minimal small talk. He would often challenge me to talk about or explore uncharted territory. He allowed me to be exactly the person I was, and I'd like to think I did the same for him.

I was able to talk with him about how my experiences shaped the way I perceived my circumstances. Soon after we met, I shared with Jamel that I had Ataxia and explained what it was. He asked me, "Do you believe you can be healed?" and I answered yes. We discussed how the way I thought about it could affect me in a positive way. We would engage in light-hearted debates about many different topics including our different and obvious experiences and viewpoints about race. It really broadened my own horizons to see how the same concept could be perceived in such dramatically different ways.

This was more than a year after separating from Sean, but heated conversations were still common between us. Jamel always encouraged me to step back and always act on whatever was in Kendall's best interest, no matter what. I wish I could say that I knew exactly why we didn't stay together. I do know that having met him and shared time together was integral to my happiness then and to my journey now. I also know that in part because of him, I continue to re-shape my own experiences and beliefs. Jamel offered me pieces of wisdom and understanding that I utilized years after we met.

Julie has been an integral character in my story for almost 20 years. On paper we are polar opposites. Sometimes our different perspectives of the same situation are like fire and ice. We grew up with dramatically different circumstances and held vastly disparate worldviews. Her entire life was spent living in various Army bases—then she joined the Army herself. She lived in Germany then returned to the States and started nursing school. We were drawn to each other's spirit, despite our lack of sameness. But as I slowly move with more unsteadiness, she is always there to reach out and provide whatever I may need. Sometimes it is more help and sometimes it is less. "I can fucking do it!" I might say, pushing her hand away, to which she says, "Good!"

> Julie,
> Thank you for being the caring friend whom I love, and I know loves me forever. For showing me that you love me unconditionally and you would do anything for me. Your belief in me and support of me has remained an aspect of our friendship that could never be replaced. We became family and will remain so, now with our beautiful children! We share a bond that was built on shared pain and loss but there is only love and fulfillment in our future.
>
> I love you, Dana

Julie and I are both suckers for "pop-up chorus." Since we're both big fans of R.E.M. too, it was a given we would go together to the Cat's Cradle in Carrboro to "just show up and sing" in April of 2015. This event was to raise money and awareness for social justice by someone who happened to have ALS. We sang "Man on the Moon," with a bunch of complete strangers and a hysterical band director. We watched the documentary about R.E.M., *Automatic Unearthed*. We had a wonderful time where we had fun while helping others.

Giving blood has proven to be a surefire way to help others in need. Trish, my friend and former teammate from Toledo, had encouraged me to give blood as a simple gesture that could make a life altering difference for someone. I had been giving whenever I could since I moved to North Carolina. Within the first few weeks of my separation from Sean, I drove by a Red Cross blood drive trailer and pulled in since I hadn't given in a while. A plastic surgery office was hosting this drive in the spring of 2012 and there happened to also be a raffle. I signed up as I was waiting for my turn. Two weeks later, they called me to tell me I won eight sessions of personal training with a local trainer, Tyrone. I would have never paid nearly $100 an hour for a personal trainer, but I was thrilled to do this free of charge.

My initial 30-minute session was so hard that when I met Julie and her two kids at the Loop that evening for a quick dinner, I was utterly exhausted. I was amazed at the strength I was able to gain and how quickly it happened: within weeks. I realized that initially I had far underestimated what I believed I could achieve. One reason for the dramatic increase in strength was that working at something that was so hard physically was also a challenge mentally. When my eight free sessions were up with Tyrone, I continued working with him for several sessions until my budget busted.

That next year I turned 40, and Ruth talked me into completing my first (and last) sprint triathlon, "The Ramblin' Rose," with her. I was pleased to have done this, but once would be enough for me. That's when I started going to Empower, a small personal training gym where Jessica was the owner. I met Jessica after her daughter had started attending at the preschool where Kendall went, right down the road from our house. I started going there to work out as they offered small group fitness classes which fit my budget much better than having a personal trainer did. I was also a fan of the types of classes they had to choose from.

During the springtime I enjoyed "Bootcamp to Beer" class where we would do an hour of boot camp–style stations outside then enjoy cold beers at the pub around the corner. The other classes I would frequent were reminiscent of my basketball days—high intensity and total body workouts. I also tried to work in Pilates or yoga occasionally or balance work on the BOSU, a half-moon-shaped inflated ball. I continued about once a week with an intense workout there and remained active in between classes for five years.

THE ATAXIAN

Every few months after I was diagnosed, I would log on to the National Ataxia Foundation website (ataxia.org) to find out what events or research studies were going on.

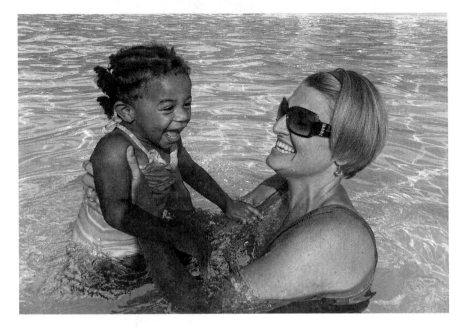

Kendall and Dana swimming at a hotel in Morrisville, North Carolina, 2010.

One of them was in 2010, when Kendall was toddling around. I took her with me to my first NAF annual meeting, which was in Chicago that year. My dad drove up from southern Indiana to join us.

We were sitting in the hallway during a break when Kendall made her way to a nearby girl about her age. She and Teagan found each other to be much more fun than the conference. Her grandmother Paula and I instantly connected. I learned that two of Paula's three daughters were there. Carli, Teagan's mom, and her younger sister Katy both had FA and were in their 20s. Sean, Kendall and I stayed at their house on a family trip to Chicago the following year. Paula and her husband host FA Woodstock each July. They invite anyone who is affected with FA to camp out for a long weekend on their farmland in northwest Indiana. They open their pool for swimming and pond for fishing, and they set up activities like making tie-dyed t-shirts. They provide the setting where people can get together to socialize and build connections that do not always come as easily for those with a rare condition.

Three years later, I was not noticeably symptomatic on the outside. On the inside, I felt incredibly aware of the many changes happening to my own abilities. In November 2014 I was working for the Center for Personalized Medicine at Duke. Christopher Austin, M.D., from the NIH came and spoke on campus about advancing translation science. My entire department was encouraged to go see his presentation as it was directly in line with our purpose. I attended with several coworkers.

Christopher P. Austin, M.D.
Director
National Center for Advancing Translational Sciences
National Institutes of Health

Christopher P. Austin, M.D., is director of the National Center for Advancing Translational Sciences (NCATS) at the National Institutes of Health (NIH). Austin leads the Center's work to improve the translation of observations in the laboratory, clinic and community into interventions that reach and benefit patients—from diagnostics and therapeutics to medical procedures and behavioral changes. Under his direction, NCATS researchers and collaborators are developing new technologies, resources and collaborative research models; demonstrating their usefulness; and disseminating the data, analysis and methodologies for use by the worldwide research community.

That night I ended up going to Tricia's house. My friend Julie had introduced me to Tricia, who was ironically now renting Ruth's old house that I had made my short-term camp-out during my initial separation from Sean. By now, I had moved back into my house in Durham and Sean had bought a house nearby in Chapel Hill, so Tricia and I were only 10 minutes apart on the same side of Durham. On nights that Kendall was staying with Sean, it wasn't uncommon for me to show up at Tricia's house, invited or not. Tricia and Julie met when they both worked in the gastrointestinal procedures unit in the hospital. They would often discuss their work, but I rarely did. Except on this night I couldn't help but talk to Tricia about the talk and the potential of "translation science."

> **Translation** is the process of turning observations in the laboratory, collating and community into interventions to improve the health of individuals in the public—from diagnostics and therapeutics to medical procedures and behavioral changes.
>
> **Translational science** is the field of investigation focused on understanding the scientific and operational principles underlying each step of the translational process.

Tricia pointed out to me how unique my own experience and perspective was. I totally agreed, but I wasn't exactly sure what I could do about it.

Three years went by and it was now April 2017. Over the days and weeks following the discussion John and I had—that it was time to write my story—thoughts and connections from my past flooded my mind constantly. In addition, over the next several months opportunities to involve myself more deeply with the cause of fighting Ataxia appeared around every corner. I discovered the Technology in Rare Neurological Disease Symposium (TRNDS). After I saw its meeting posted on the NAF's Facebook page, I immediately registered to attend and booked my flight to Rochester on May 12, 2017. This was a luxury that I wasn't used to—being available to go somewhere at the drop of a hat, but I could because I was no longer working.

During a break in the meeting mid-morning, I called the National Ataxia Foundation and Sue Hagan answered. I could hardly contain my excitement after hearing the speakers and what they were saying. More than 25 experts in their fields had shown up to participate in a discussion of how what they do could contribute to the field of advancing therapeutics for rare neurological disorders. At the end of the meeting I had taken five pages of barely legible notes, since my handwriting has gotten progressively worse over the last several years due to Ataxia. I have devised my own version of "shorthand" that requires the least amount of writing but contains keywords that are meaningful to me. By no means was I trying to document everything that was discussed, only capture the items that were truly meaningful to me. These notes would be put to good use. A few days after I returned home, Sue Hagen asked me if I would be willing to write up a summary of the meeting for the NAF patient newsletter, and with John's guidance, I did.

There was going to be a local Ataxia support group meeting on April 22, 2017, in nearby Garner. I emailed the organizer, Ron, and confirmed that I would be at the meeting. When I arrived, Ron introduced the guest speaker who would be talking about yoga for people with disabilities. Then he introduced a special guest who just happened to be in town that day. It was Joel Sutherland, the executive director of the National Ataxia Foundation (NAF). He spoke for only a few minutes, but I was immediately drawn to his personality and his energy. He mentioned to the small group that it would be great to find people that could raise money locally to help fund more research.

I immediately raised my hand and said, "I need to talk to you before you leave." When we broke for lunch, I introduced myself and told him that I would help raise money for NAF. He gave me his card to email him, and he took off to go catch his flight back to Minnesota. Over the next eight weeks I picked up the phone and called friends and relatives, messaged, emailed, and posted on Facebook consistently up through June 2017. Friends, family and complete strangers donated to the National Ataxia Foundation.

On my way to the Ataxia support meeting in Garner I tested a Cat Trike, a low-riding three-wheeled racing bike like Kyle Bryant rode in the documentary *The Ataxian*. *The Ataxian* features Kyle and Sean Baumstark, both suffering from different stages of Friedreich's Ataxia (FA) and led an incredible cross-country journey across America on their bikes in 2010. I was aware of the documentary since 2015 and I had been trying but failing to go see it when it was being screened. It was finally released in February 2018 and I watched it on Amazon in early March at my house. It was one of the most moving documentaries I have ever seen. Kyle is a shining

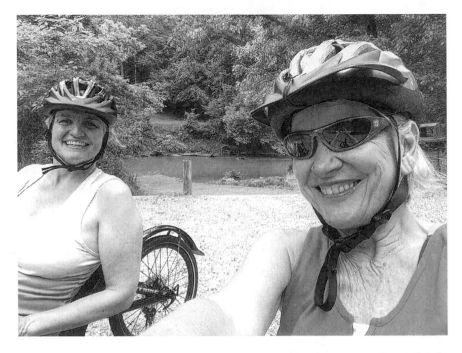

Dana Creighton (left) and Shirley Kunkel on Falls of Neuse trail in Raleigh, North Carolina, 2017.

star for raising awareness for FA and inspiring hope by the way he chooses to live. I transitioned to my own funky new three-wheeled bike just a few weeks after my test drive.

The money from the sale of my traditional bike was donated to my NAF fundraising campaign. I had several encounters that helped bring out my own desire to help. One of the many things I had mastered in my career was diving in headfirst to get exactly what I was looking for. In 2014, I sent Kyle Bryant a message on Facebook asking him about his thoughts on intense exercise and Ataxia. This was before I had heard about his documentary, *The Ataxian*. I knew who he was as he had been a guest speaker at the NAF meeting in Chicago talking about his experiences with adaptive fitness. Three years later, I reached out to Sean Baumstark, Kyle's partner on their trek across America in *The Ataxian*. I cold-called Sean and introduced myself to him to get his perspective on what he felt needed to be done. Sean told me about the upcoming FDA meeting in a few weeks, June 2, 2017, in College Park, Maryland.

This would be a full day where Friedreich's Ataxia Research Alliance (FARA) and hundreds of patients and families would get a chance to tell the FDA why finding a treatment and cure for FA is so imperative. Sean invited me to come to this meeting. I wanted and needed to be there and learn from this subset of Ataxians. Everyone that spoke told stories of how their lives were affected by FA. Some had family members who were already gone, others were recently diagnosed and everything in between. Personal and scientific stories were told all day and the energy in the room was palpable and incredibly hopeful. Ron Bartek, who founded Friedreich's Ataxia Research Alliance (FARA) in 1998, told his own personal journey. They have established and built a strong research alliance by investing in their own patients' well-being and listening to what drives them in their search for a treatment together as one unit.

After the meeting I introduced myself to Ron Bartek and told him how inspiring his story was to me. I heard it for the first time that day. A few weeks later when I saw him again, unexpectedly in Bethesda at the NCATS Smarter Science meeting, he gave me a huge bear hug and an enormous kiss on the cheek like we were long lost cousins. I had found my people and my purpose. Now it was becoming clearer to me what I could do to help. I could help align and connect people who could move forward advancements in Ataxia research.

CHAPTER V

No Longer Asking Why

Is there an answer to the question of why bad things happen to good people? The response would be ... to forgive the world for not being perfect, to forgive God for not making a better world, to reach out to the people around us, and to go on living despite it all ... no longer asking why something happened, but asking how we will respond, what we intend to do now that it has happened.
—Harold S. Kushner

EMPOWERED

I fractured my sacrum in June 2017, which put me out of commission for a solid six weeks. There is no treatment regimen to speed up or heal a broken back. Time and rest is the prescription. Finally, I was physically healed enough to start exercising again. I signed up for a group fitness class at Empower and during the first five minutes it was apparent to me that my training hiatus had strongly impacted my strength and especially my balance. I cautiously finished the rest of the class. My experience working individually with a personal trainer had been a wake-up call that my life as an athlete could be recreated, at least on a small scale until I regained my strength and confidence. I decided that now was the time to work with a trainer again. I chose Nestor to be my personal trainer.

Nestor was in the final treatments of his two-year-long battle with a brain tumor, which included brain surgery, chemotherapy and radiation. My first training session with Nestor was more for him to size me up and determine what his plan would be for me. I recall that it was relatively easy to do each exercise he had me perform, but that as I held my grip and my entire body weight while performing lateral pull ups, my fear of falling and reinjuring my back rose to the forefront of my mind. I also realized that because the exercises were at a basic level I could focus my energy on reminding my body how to reestablish the brain to muscle pathways of these movements.

As the weeks passed, the workouts got progressively harder and more complex. He eventually introduced me to the crab walk and the bear walk (down and back forward and backward) was absolute hell, but doable. Nestor had applied his knowledge of strength training and utilized his own personal connection with a brain injury to develop a personalized and unique program that would stretch the limits of my own abilities. Part of maintaining a sense of normalcy with a progressive condition that doesn't slow down and wait is to continue to do things that give you joy.

One day Nestor had me cooling down shooting baskets on a seven-foot rim using a kid's ball. I was coordinating my lower body with my upper body and I was utilizing hand-eye coordination. After just a couple of minutes of fumbling, I locked into making most of my shots. And I was recruiting muscles and a brain that had decades of experience to help. As time goes on, I am physically less able to do exercises that require balance and coordination. I still challenge my body and mind to do as much as they can.

Exercise is for me a re-calibration of my mind-body connection. If you don't consistently calibrate the equipment it will get farther and farther away from the intended target. Mine is optimal well-being on a sliding scale. *The Brain That Changes Itself* had no doubt been a game changer in how I thought about having Ataxia. Based on my genetics, I was bound to someday become symptomatic. I also had four decades of training—physically, mentally, emotionally, and spiritually. Michele Vincenzo Malacarne proposed

> that neural tissue might respond to exercise as do muscles. Malacarne set out to test Bonnet's hypothesis experimentally. He took pairs of birds that came from the same clutch of eggs and raised half of them

under enriched circumstances, stimulated by intensive training for several years. The other half received no training. He did the same experiment to littermate dogs. When he sacrificed the animals and compared the brain size, he found that the animals that received training had larger brains, particularly in that part of the brain called the cerebellum, demonstrating the influence of "enriched circumstances" and "training" on the development of the individual's brain [315].

With my own training in exercise physiology and my intimate knowledge of how my body was responding to different stimuli, I decided it was time to start training myself. The night before I went to the gym on my own to work out, I was rereading a portion of Norman Doidge's book about the different types of neuroplasticity. The brain can adapt and make accommodations to changing situations in multiple ways. As I was warming up on the elliptical machine, I was thinking about this, not associating it with my workout. Then I realized that I was watching myself in the mirror across the room and that it was likely a benefit to my brain to visually see myself moving in such a smooth and coordinated way, reinforcing the exercise not just with my muscles and nervous system but also in the visual cortex of my brain.

I thought of myself as a car as it gets older. My engine becomes increasingly less efficient, but that doesn't bother me as I'm still the one in control of where I am going.

I had been meeting with John for a year now. John knew of my history with Dr. Tom Clouse and it had been years since our last correspondence. He encouraged me to reach out to him again, so I did in early March 2017.

> Tom,
>
> OK, so in a nutshell over the past 10 years, my symptoms are progressing as of course I expected. About 5 years ago I won 8 free sessions with a personal trainer. I ended up really amazing myself and increasing my overall strength, fitness and confidence. I no longer work with a trainer, but exercise regularly (only about once a week intensely). I still ride my bike and will more now that spring is near. And really there is nothing I cannot do (although there are a lot of things that I don't do very well). I also reduced my hours from 40 to 30

hours a week of work about 5 years ago. My bottom line now is that I feel like I need to do something that will benefit the Ataxia community.

I have also seen a physical therapist (PT) a few times in the last 5 years, and I incorporate these highly specific coordination and balance training exercises into my weekly routine.

So, I am asking you that based on your interactions with many and ongoing patients, where do you see the need for action?

Dana

Dana,

That is great in what you have found and what you now know you must continue doing. "What works" for you to keep your movement abilities as natural and normal as possible, and what works for you to maintain your "normal as anyone else" lifestyle, is not mysterious or magical. What works for you is what you have learned you need to do with your situation. It works because you are not living the label that others want to throw on you and restrict you to. It works because you realized that you have choices regardless of what your "order" inside may be. It works because you are using common sense to find your truth within yourself.

Dana, was it the PT and the Trainer that provided you with these things? No. They were a tool and resource to help and support you to find it on your own.

Tom

Although I was still working at Duke, Dr. Clouse's response to me tipped the momentum that took me into new and uncharted territory. I started organizing the dozens of medical records, scientific articles, and personal notes I had been saving all of my life. Back in graduate school in 1999 I requested and then received from IU Medical Center several pages of medical records mostly from my Grandpa Earl and his daughter Carolyn and son Bill. His brothers Bob and Dave were seen by different institutions but information about each of them was documented in Carolyn's record. IU Medical Center had a typewritten document that my mother had made to describe the pedigree in written form. This included who was affected with her estimation of when symptoms first appeared in the entire Poynter family, written on her typewriter around 1983.

My mom's documentation of who was affected and at what age

their symptoms began somehow landed in Carolyn's medical record years after she was deceased. My grandma Lorene had a classmate from school that she remained friends with throughout her life. My cousin Vickie had filled me in on this connection and said everyone on her side of the family referred to Lorene as Granny. This friend of Granny's happened to have a son who was getting his doctorate in medical genetics and recorded Carolyn's family history at IU Medical Center in 1974. Maybe this was how new information was landing in medical records post-mortem. Granny may have been the mule trafficking information that my mom was orchestrating in the early 1980s.

Stop Fighting

There are moments in life when time seems to stop momentarily, and a realization sets in. The moment happened in 2017 when I was home alone one evening. I had been divorced from Sean for more than five years and Kendall was staying at his house that night. I stumbled upon the *TED Radio Hour* on NPR on my laptop, a series of short segments of TED talks making up a one-hour program titled *Maslow's Hierarchy of Needs*. Carolyn Casey had been legally blind her entire life and at 27 she had worked her way across several different professions. She finally got tired of pretending to be someone else and said, "I need help."

> "Why are you trying so hard *not* to be yourself?" her eye doctor asked. He then said, "Do you love your job; do you love what you do? I think it's time to stop fighting and do something different."

This resonated with me deeply. I had always been a hard worker, but I was putting intense effort into camouflaging my movements and displaying to others that it was all under control. I was still working 30 hours a week in health research. My condition was progressive so now in my early 40s I was dealing with steadily increasing symptoms. When I heard Carolyn say those words—"I need help"—I felt a visceral release as I sobbed, imagining what it would be like if I could actually say those words too.

For months I had been aggressively looking for another job and frequently visited the human resources website. This day the lead article on the HR homepage was about the Office of Disability Management. I was not familiar with this department, so I read about its services and I called the office. I described how I had been diagnosed with a progressive neurological disorder in 2006 and how I took a Family Medical Leave of Absence (FMLA) in late 2011 after working and quickly becoming overwhelmed in a new department. After returning from my short hiatus in 2012, I returned to the same department I had just left a few weeks prior and remained there for five years.

We discussed what they did, and it seemed to fit what I needed, which was to ensure job security despite my condition. I was talking to one of the directors and she swiftly recommended that I contact someone who handles accommodation requests. After I got off the phone, I contacted her and immediately started the process. I completed an accommodation request with a doctor on staff and this was forwarded to my supervisor. As much as I had been resisting the possibility of reaching out for help, it wasn't long before I fully gave in to the notion that it was time to stop pretending that I was fine and make a change.

The alternative was to find and secure another similar-level position. I had already found out firsthand that if you are being paid a certain salary, no department is interested in hiring you into a lower-level position and be forced to pay your current salary. I was already living as my authentic self with my best friends, all our children and my entire family. It was time to admit that I needed help and give up the career that lent itself to having me conceal my weaknesses and forge ahead as if nothing was wrong. Then, about a week later, my supervisor walked in and gave me official notice that my position would end. The funding would be ending so my position would no longer be available. I quickly called the doctor I had been working with to prepare paperwork for my accommodation request. He suggested we meet first thing the next morning in his office.

When I arrived early to our appointment the next day the office staff said he didn't come into the office on Thursdays. This was my first clue that there was an urgency for him to speak with me. When he did call me in to his office, he quickly got to the point that clearly my intention to put accommodations in place were meant to be protective to my position. But the day my current position ended I would not be eligible to receive *any* accommodations. On top of that, I would need to secure a new position within the next 60 days and most likely at 40 hours per week, not 30 which I had become accustomed to for the previous five years. Then I would need to be offered the job and hired, and then I would have to present my accommodation request to that new department. They would then have the right to say that they could or could not work with the requested accommodations.

I was realizing that moving into another position had the potential to create an environment that could be detrimental to my physical and mental health which as I was getting older was of the highest importance to me—in order to be a mom. And although my current department did not know my entire backstory, it had proven to be flexible and accommodating to my situation. Then he very kindly stated that although he was sure it was not my intention to go down the road leading to disability, I must seriously consider this as an option and consider it very soon or not at all. Once I was no longer employed, I was no longer eligible for this benefit.

I informed my best friend of nearly 20 years, Julie, that I was going to apply for disability and leave my job. We met years before I was diagnosed, and she had proven to be one of my biggest advocates. She had been suggesting I consider this for the past several months. I always outright rejected her suggestion, as I cringed in horror at the thought. I explained to her further that after I applied for disability, if my request was denied, I had made the decision to not return to work again, period. Her reaction was just short of "Have you lost your mind?" The answer was no, I was fully prepared for the possibility that there was no guarantee, as my neurologist and therapist reminded me. So I went out of work on FMLA leave in April of 2017 as I had done before in 2011. I completed all the paperwork required for employer disability as well as worked up a financial plan with my brother Brian, who had a degree in finance, based on if I got approved for disability or if I didn't.

It was the last week of March 2017 and it was my daughter's spring break. I had accrued plenty of vacation time. This helped me make the decision to take the week of spring break off to be with her. We drove four hours west to Asheville, North Carolina, and stayed in a bed and breakfast that was close enough to downtown that we could walk there each day. The weather was nice, and we would explore different ways to walk to the eclectic stores and restaurants. We had the TV on in our room one morning and I saw a family being interviewed on a national morning news show.

The Demoes' story felt so close to my own family that it was hard for me to believe it was not fiction. They suffered from a form of Alzheimer's disease that has the same hereditary pattern as my family and strikes much younger than the typical form. Their story is chronicled in *The Inheritance: A Family on the Front Lines of the Battle Against Alzheimer's Disease* by Niki Kapsambelis. When I got back to Durham, I ordered it online and read it. Out of all the books I had read over the past several years, I had never identified as closely as I did with *The Inheritance*. It became possible for me to think about my own life in story form. I was fascinated by how the story flowed between the family's personal narrative and their struggle with the inherited form of Alzheimer's disease and their ongoing quest to help move science forward in hope of finding a treatment or cure.

> In February 2004, Gail received a disturbingly familiar phone call from a coworker of Brian and Doug. "Gail, I think there's something wrong with your boys," he confessed. "They aren't able to do their jobs like they were." The news didn't come as a complete surprise; for a few months, the family had been making the same observation. Since his late 20s, Doug—who, ironically, shared a birthday with his uncle Jerry—had been repeating himself. And while everybody in town noticed it, nobody wanted to believe the disease was coming back for

another round. But fear was beginning to simmer in their collective subconscious [*The Inheritance* 104].

I had been reading more and more since my divorce in 2012 and almost exclusively non-fiction. I didn't choose books that I felt resembled my story. I did the opposite—I chose authors with wildly different backgrounds, from Eminem and Patti Smith to Sidney Poitier and Sonia Sotomayor. I read dozens of memoirs, from both well-known and not well-known authors. It was when John suggested that I read *Writing Hard Stories: Celebrated Memoirists Who Shaped Art from Trauma* by Melanie Brooks that I felt compelled to not only write but share my story.

> This is what I want, I thought. I want my father's story, *my story*, to be something other than this crushing weight of grief that I carry so close. I want it to be something different. Something meaningful. But my fear of really examining that grief is standing in my way [*Writing Hard Stories* 5].

I had been meeting with John for a full year now, and suddenly the path had been cleared in my mind and I began to outline my story.

Adjusting the Focus

As soon as I filed for FMLA in April 2017, I was no longer required to work. During this time, I had a conversation with John about how I really wanted to compare the trajectory of my symptoms of Ataxia with my exercise type and intensity over the last 10 years. Thinking about this along with sketching out a simple diagram triggered my brain to also think about how an individual's repeat number correlates to age of onset and speed of progression. I also had access to my very own geneticist, Dr. Tom Kunkel. Tom and his wife Shirley lived in my neighborhood but on another street. Tom was a research scientist with a Ph.D. in genetics, and he ran a laboratory and had done research at National

Institute of Environmental Health Sciences (NIEHS) for more than 30 years.

We had lived in the same neighborhood for eight years without ever crossing paths for long enough to introduce ourselves. That changed after we brought Kendall home in 2008. Sean and I, who typically walked our three dogs around the neighborhood, now also took Kendall in her stroller. Tom and Shirley are not ones to see a new baby and not introduce themselves and share just a little in the new joy and excitement. It's hard to recall not knowing them now. They were instantly a part of our extended family as Shirley gleefully offered to help whenever we needed it. She did, and she still does for Sean and me.

I posed a question to Tom on one of my usual and frequent visits to their house.

> How does an individual's repeat number [derived from measurable information from DNA at the mutation location] correlate to age of onset and speed of progression?

Tom is the head of the DNA replication group and does not do clinical research in humans. He encouraged me to investigate this further since this was not his area of expertise.

Repeat number is solely diagnostic and can broadly determine severity (in SCA2 repeats above 100 are likely to result in symptoms in infancy and just above 35 can result in a later onset), but there are clearly other factors at play. Epigenetic changes as well as genetic factors may influence the expression of the repeat. As I found out when I read *The Inheritance*, identical twin sisters Julia and Agnes Noonan had early onset Alzheimer's, but their age of onset was more than a decade apart.

> As identical twins, they shared the same genome, including their genetic mutation. But because their lifespans differed significantly, researchers later theorized the difference in their disease progression may have been epigenetic caused by outside factors that modify the genome and change the pattern of how genes are expressed without changing the actual DNA sequence. Diet and environmental factors, for example, can create epigenetic changes [117].

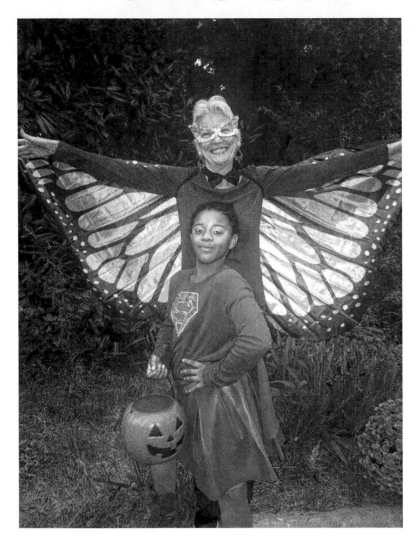

Shirley Kunkel and Kendall, Durham, North Carolina, Halloween, 2016. Shirley helped make Kendall's costume.

The genetic variation expressed by two different presentations occurring in twins is as controlled as we are likely to get. My first cousins Susie and Betsy both died at age 35 in 1991 and in 1995. At the time, I was totally unaware of their deaths and I had never even met Susie. I can remember one visit from Betsy, who was already in a wheelchair, at our farmhouse with her older sister Marti when I was a freshman in high school. Betsy talked a lot and appeared very happy and joyful as I thought to myself, "How could anyone with her condition not be absolutely devastated by it?" She clearly was not, and although her speech was significantly affected, she chatted away about her activities with the church.

Todd, Scott and I each had an age of onset later and speed of progression that was slower than our first cousins.

1. Possibly from inheriting a balance of DNA from both sets of grandparents, which might have had some protective qualities.
2. Or because the mutation Mom passed on to us was not as severe as the mutation her siblings passed to their children.
3. Or some of each, along with other factors, including each with a rate of progression that may or may not have been also preprogrammed.

For SCA2, a repeat value of over 32 = affected

Mom/deceased	no test available (affected)
Todd	never tested (affected)
Brian	22 repeats (not affected)
Scott/deceased	44 repeats (affected)
Dana	43 repeats (affected)

My mom was the only one of the five siblings who had more than one affected child, so there are no other scenarios within her family to make comparisons with. If my brothers and I sat down to play a game of Uno, played with our genetic dice—Todd, Scott, and Dana drew a "wild card" on our first turn, all three with an age of onset that may or may not have been preprogrammed in our DNA. Lucky for Brian, after Todd drew his wild card, he drew a skip card. But we all four would make the lives we had by how we shaped our own realities.

CHEERS

My brain was running on overdrive on this story that was slowly taking shape. Talking with my neighbor Tom was energizing my quest to continue going down unknown paths. Kendall had joined Shirley at the strawberry patch each spring since she was a toddler. They would join Tom and everyone in his lab to pick berries. Shirley and Tom would take them home and clean them so the next day everyone would convene in a conference room to enjoy the annual "Strawberry Feast"—shortcake with whipped cream, ice cream, chocolate for dipping, and many other possible ways to consume them.

Every spring while I was still working, Shirley offered to pick Kendall up from elementary school and head out to the lab in Research Triangle Park. Since I was not working this year, it was my first time attending with them instead of hearing about it second-hand. When we arrived, everyone was already eating, talking and enjoying the desserts. Shirley knew many of the attendees and even Kendall knew the other kids from attending lab parties with the Kunkels for years. It was no surprise to me that I would be enjoying my treats by myself. As a textbook introvert, keeping to myself in these settings is highly preferred over chatting up unknown partygoers.

So I was happily ingesting my strawberries when the two women I was seated next to appeared to have finished their in-depth conversation, likely about their work. The woman directly to my right, assuming I belonged somewhere in the institute, asked me what lab I worked in. I chuckled and said, "No, no I'm just here with Shirley—who is married to Tom Kunkel." I asked her what she did there, and she replied that she looked at mechanisms of DNA repair. I told her that I had a very primitive and basic knowledge of genetics. "What does this mean practically?" She went on to explain a little more and she used the term "trinucleotide repeat expansions." I frantically raised my hand and said, "Oh, oh, that's me!" She replied, "Cool!"

We continued talking and exchanged contact information. Her name was Phyllis Strauss and she was a professor at Northeastern

University in Boston. She was in Durham for eight weeks as a visiting professor, doing research with another lab at NIEHS, where my neighbor Tom had spent most of his career. We met for coffee and lunch a few times at Guglhupf, a delicious German bakery in Durham, and we talked through the science of my kind of disorder and what her theories were about how to repair them. I have a pretty good handle on basic science and genetics, but it was a little like Frasier Crane explaining psychoanalytic concepts to Woody Boyd.

She mentioned just a couple of different modulations that may affect the expression of the static genome. One was the potential impact of nutrition—the example she gave was of relatively short-term changes potentially changing not only the expression of offspring but *their* offspring as well. The other example forced me to think in terms of not only *how my repeat number determines my outcome*, but what else can the sum of *all of my genetic material NOT associated with the mutation* account for? Phyllis returned to Boston that fall, but we have kept in touch. Here is a correspondence shortly after she returned home.

Hi Dana,

Your original question to me was:

Is it possible that genetic variation of disease expression of different markers (not at the mutation location) that have been passed to affected person by non-affected parent be a factor in determining their gene expression (and not be reflected in repeat number)?

Complicated, isn't it! I'm sure that your dad's genome might cause modifications with sibs. Have you ever looked into the lives of your grandparents?

Also, nutritional factors might cause modulations of the identical sequence. There are some interesting starvation studies that indicate this possibility. They were not done on purpose, but during WWII the Nazis cut off food supplies to the north of Holland from the south. Then the canals froze, and it was not possible to move foodstuffs to the north. Lots of people died of starvation. Children who were in utero at the time had a higher incidence of diabetes and obesity later. What was most interesting is that THEIR children also had metabolism problems.

Anyway, greetings from Boston. The weather here is crisp and cool, which I just love. Enough with the North Carolina stuff!

Phyllis

I was originally reading *It Didn't Start with You* in the context of inherited family trauma. The picture that Mark Wolynn paints below transformed my own interpretation of what *genetically inherited* can encompass.

> ... before your mother was even born, your mother, your grandmother, and the earliest traces of you were all in the same body—three generations sharing the same biological environment. This isn't a new idea: embryology textbooks have told us as much for more than a century. Your inception can be similarly traced in your terminal line. The precursor cells of the sperm you developed from present in your father when he was a fetus in his mother's womb [25–26].

Our meetings while she was here and our continued correspondence helped me understand what other factors may be influencing age of onset and progression that I had never considered—like the many factors which may influence how different genes are expressed, like nutrition and the combination of genes inherited by four different grandparents.

SHEER FANTASY

In my brother Scott's obituary, my dad directed contributions be made to Stefan Pulst's lab. I had already been following the work of Dr. Stefan Pulst at the University of Utah. My dad, a biology teacher for 30 years, was also hopeful that what he was doing was novel and promising. Phyllis also sent me these results from Stefan Pulst's recent and encouraging ASO therapy, performed in mice. Modified antisense oligonucleotides (ASOs) provide a unique tool to target mRNA transcripts in vivo.

Degenerative Ataxias, from genes to therapies: The 2015 Cotzias
   Lecture.
Pulst, S.M. *Neurology*. 2016 Jun 14; 86(24): 2284–90.

It can take more than a decade to go from a proposed model of a potential therapy to testing in humans. First, it is tested in mice to see if the proposed therapy even works as you have proposed it would. The next step, testing in humans, is usually years away. Hopefully, this will be a look into the future and this ASO therapy will help defend against many debilitating conditions.

ASO Therapy: Hope for Genetic Neurological Diseases
Muth, C.C., M.D. *JAMA*. 2018; 319(7): 644–646.

In 2016, new therapies for spinal muscular atrophy (SMA) and Duchenne muscular dystrophy (DMD), neuromuscular diseases caused by rare genetic mutations, were approved by the US Food and Drug Administration. Characterized by progressive muscle weakness and premature death, these diseases are devastating; in the most severe type of SMA, for example, children are unable to sit or stand unassisted and typically die before 2 years of age due to respiratory muscle weakness.

...The recently approved treatments, nusinersen for SMA and eteplirsen for DMD, share a common therapeutic approach: the use of antisense oligonucleotides (ASOs).

...In a recent trial involving 122 infants with SMA, 51% of children who received nusinersen demonstrated improvement in motor milestones (for some this included the ability to roll over, sit independently, or stand), compared with none of the children who received placebo.

Studies like this offer genuine hope that certain research models will make a purposeful difference to people of all ages. I attended the 62nd National Ataxia Conference in Las Vegas in 2019, "Ataxia: A Treatable Disease," since there are multiple ways that we can defend against Ataxia including adapting to diminishing abilities with dignity. Back at the conference in 2017, I had learned about a specific piece of this whole puzzle that I was never aware of. It gave me a new perspective on the minds of the doctors that had been advising Mom for more than ten years. The doctors in the 1970s and 1980s only knew that the symptoms of inherited Ataxias tended to be similar by generation. And since three of Mom's siblings were symptomatic by or in their 20s doctors arrived at the erroneous assumption that she had likely escaped the same fate. Ataxia is now known to be a *trinucleotide repeat expansion disorder.* These disorders are also now known to be affected by genetic anticipation.

Chapter V. No Longer Asking Why

> Anticipation in genetics—subsequent generations are likely to be affected
> at an earlier age of onset (with likely faster progression of degeneration)
> of the parent from whom the condition was inherited from.

The full scope of how anticipation affects a condition and what sequence caused this mutation was not illuminated until well into the 1990s. Different doctors were hedging their bets for my mom for good reason. The limited evidence they had at the time did not warrant crisis intervention for Mom—it warranted a hope and a prayer. *Being Mortal* is a book written by Dr. Atul Gawande that I had wanted to read for almost a year. The content of the book always seemed too heavy for me to dive into, so I happily put it off. I was at church early in 2018 and the service bulletin listed that the documentary *Being Mortal* was going to be shown in the fellowship hall the following Wednesday. Yay for documentaries! This was now in fact very pertinent, as my dad, almost 78, was in the midst of excruciating pain in most of his joints for several weeks. My brother Todd, at 55, was nearing the end of his course of his solitary and semi-independent living in his home. My dad was his primary caregiver, so my brother Brian spent almost a month helping them both daily in different households.

I was riveted by the documentary and what Dr. Gawande revealed inspired me to immediately borrow the book from my friend Tricia. Sara Thomas Monopoli was just 34 and pregnant with her first child when doctors learned she was going to die. Instead of an infection, as everyone had expected, she had lung cancer and it had already spread to the lining in her chest.

> Step-by-step, Sarah ended up on a fourth-round chemotherapy, one
> with the minuscule likelihood of altering the course of her disease and
> the great likelihood of causing debilitating side effects. An opportunity
> to prepare for the inevitable was forgone. It all happened because of an
> assuredly normal circumstance: a patient and family unready to con-
> front the reality of her disease [*Being Mortal* 167].

Not only stage IV lung cancer but now thyroid cancer was ravaging through her body.

After one of her chemotherapies seemed to shrink the thyroid cancer slightly, I even raised with her the possibility that an experimental therapy could work against both her cancers, which was sheer fantasy. Discussing a fantasy was easier—less emotional, less explosive, less prone to misunderstanding than discussing what was happening before my eyes [169].

It was at that moment I no longer held the doctors accountable for delivering news to Mom that altered her perception of her risk. Doctor and patient relationships rely on each other to add integral pieces shared from both parties. Honest and sometimes difficult scenarios allow both sides to understand the possible implications of each. As with life, sometimes we can be a part of something doctors never could have predicted. My friend Randy and his wife Elaine tried for seven years to get pregnant. Doctors finally told them that use of medications for so long had thinned the lining in Elaine's uterus enough that pregnancy was no longer a viable option. The couple then had two children over the next five years.

After the PGD debacle, Sean and I transferred our remaining frozen embryos to a facility much closer to us. When Kendall was an infant, we tried without success at pregnancy. Even if our hope is lost, others may still find theirs. It wasn't until the annual NAF meeting that I attended in Philadelphia in 2018 that I heard about the stories of three mothers with Ataxia who had a grand total of seven children, from newborns to age 14, through this process of PGD. I'm sure there were more, but I heard the personal stories of these three women, one directly and two indirectly through conversations.

SEEDS OF FEAR

My dad's family provided their ongoing support to us. It was 1988 and I had not spent much time with my dad's mother recently. She had been diagnosed with Alzheimer's disease. I was a freshman on the high school volleyball team when my dad arrived early to pick me up from practice. He told me that my grandma, his mother Helen, had just driven her car into Center Lake and had taken her own life. She was a strong and steady presence in my life. She was very pleasant and loving and I admired her. She had played on an intramural basketball team in the 1920s and played golf her entire adult life.

In my 20s, my dad pointed out to me that when I drove, I tapped my thumbs to the music while holding the steering wheel, exactly like his mom used to do. Then, and still today, I do this instinctively, without thinking. I tried to explain that maybe it was a learned habit I acquired from watching her. I can remember riding in the car with her when I was little, but only occasionally. If it was learned, then that was a powerful bit of a useless behavior that was imprinted on my brain though it would be years before I could utilize it. Maybe I shared more than I could have ever realized with my ancestors from both sides of the family.

Kendall had just finished third grade in 2017 and my dad was driving on our trip through Yellowstone National Park.

I was in the passenger seat and cringed when we were driving around corners with deep cliffs to my right. I told Dad that I had recently found a picture on the Internet of Earl Poynter, my mom's father, when he was in high school. He told me as an adult, Earl was deathly afraid of going over bridges. Later he commented that Mom could not ride in the passenger seat when she faced directly over a steep canyon when we were in Yellowstone as a family in 1978. She had to go in the back of the camper. My dad then told me, "You know that your fear is associated with Ataxia" (since my mom and her dad both had this condition as well as the fear). I told him, "No, it isn't"—I believe that it may be "inherited family trauma" and was *not definitely* "related to Ataxia."

> What I've learned from my own experience, training, and clinical practice is the answer may not lie within our own story as much as in the stories of our parents, grandparents and even our great grandparents. The latest scientific research, now making headlines, also tells us that

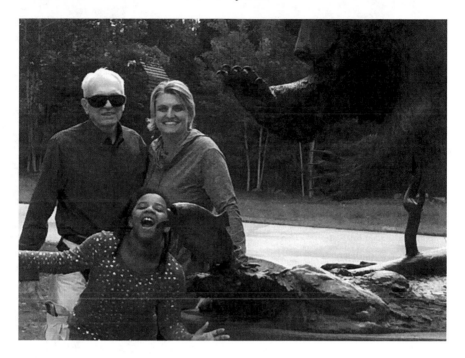

Robert and Dana Creighton and Kendall on summer vacation in Yellowstone National Park, Wyoming, 2017.

the effects of trauma can pass from one generation to the next. This "bequest" is what's known as inherited family trauma, and emerging evidence suggests that it is a very real phenomenon.

Pain does not always dissolve on its own or diminish with time. Even if the person who suffered the original trauma has died, even if his or her story lies submerged in years, fragments of life experience, memory, and body sensation can live on, as if reaching out from the past to find resolution in the minds and bodies of those living in the present [*It Didn't Start with You* 1].

As a child, my brother Scott was terrified of loud noises. When Scott was three, Dad carried him to the car with his hands pressed tightly over his ears, crying while watching the fireworks display in nearby Akron. When I asked my dad about this, he commented that he used to react to loud noises in the same panicked way as Scott when he was young. This is not proof of inherited family trauma. For me, it signifies a real possibility that the overwhelming fear my mother and brother exhibited was not strictly dependent on their circumstances surrounding Ataxia, but a combination of that with a deep-seated fear that felt outside of their control.

> A newborn baby has only two basic fears, the fear of falling and the fear of sudden loud noises. These are perfectly normal. They serve as a sort of alarm system given to you by nature as a means of self-preservation.
>
> Normal fear is good. You hear an automobile coming down the road and you step aside to survive. The momentary fear of being run over is overcome by your action.
>
> All other fears are abnormal. They were caused by a particular experience or were passed along to you by parents, relatives, teachers, and others who influenced your early years [*The Power of Your Subconscious Mind* 248].

I can remember a conversation Scott and I had when we were roughly 12 and 13 years old in the kitchen at the farmhouse. We decided it would be best to live our lives assuming that someday we would in fact be diagnosed with the condition. We both found it hard to swallow that we could go through our life thinking we would not get it, only to be blindsided if we did develop the condition at some point—like Mom had. I believe that throughout her entire adult life, my mom dreaded the possibility of a positive diagnosis. Her fear of having a strong chance of getting the disease had been increasing throughout the 1960s, when she already had two young children. Then Mom and Dad went to the Mayo Clinic in 1971, when Dr. Hymie Gordon told her that she had only about a 10 percent chance of getting it. This prognosis was given with only her best interest in mind, although it was certainly not congruent with a dominantly inherited condition, which had already been firmly established.

The correspondence Mom saved about how things happened within her family and medical professionals she saw was like a trail she left that I followed. However small, she did have a tiny amount of hope—or why methodically save this information in the first place? She started saving letters before I was born. So she didn't save them for me, but when my dad passed the baton to me in 1998, I utilized them to help me understand how her story progressed. And the connection with my mom that I wanted desperately my entire life was now happening 25 years after her death.

One of my mom's hobbies she enjoyed before her diagnosis was doing puzzles. I remember this clearly when we lived in the Southbrook Park house. This was also something that was included on the growing list of things she gave up in the years following her diagnosis. Another thing she unknowingly gave up was trying to figure out how the pieces of her life went together. The pieces had became so foreign and misshapen. It was as if the picture on the box had been erased and she was left to make the pieces fit together with no guidance to help her figure out how it should look.

I was at Julie's house on a recent Labor Day weekend and writing furiously. She was just one day post-op from major surgery and was in recovery mode. She had ordered a puzzle ahead of time, knowing she should do as little as possible during her recovery. She was just beginning the 1000-piece puzzle. It appeared to me to be virtually impossible—a beautiful scene of a landscape in Paris. All morning she worked on the puzzle and she had not yet completed the straight edges after three hours of tedious work. Later that day I was thinking that her framing the edges of the puzzle was like me writing down my story. Beginning to write about my life experiences was a gateway to figuring out how the pieces of my life fit together. Without the outer framework being done, there was little hope that the bigger picture would reveal itself.

Sean and I have been divorced for almost 10 years. I was horrified to admit to my dad that we were going to separate. What I feared the most was stuck in my mind only. My dad immediately offered his full support to me. Time after time I have been reminded that facing fear usually involves the worst-case scenario. What plays out in real time has no choice but to be affected by how I choose to react to those circumstances. Unlike my mom, I grew up with an awareness of the malady that ran in our family. From a young age I very consciously chose a path that was inverse to Mom's. Her path had been blazed subconsciously by fear for years.

The seeds of fear are planted in all of our minds, in one way or another. Finding a strategy to hone in on what coping mechanism to rid the fear for you is highly individualized. Religion is a type of coping mechanism, I would argue. Focusing your faith and energy on God's will and living a life that is driven by the Almighty is favored by many, as opposed to letting the seeds of fear flourish in the fertile ground of the plastic brain, conforming and contorting a potentially horrific story of where your circumstances will lead you.

FRANKENSTEIN

The neurologic pathology in my family had different presentations. My brother Scott, who was only a year and a half older than me, had been symptomatic since his mid–20s. His repeat number was only one up from mine but our Ataxia journeys were miles apart. Todd, who was eight years older, had shown symptoms in his 20s too, but Scott was progressing at a more rapid pace. Scott was a free spirit and liked to philosophize about politics and the economy, was multilingual, traveled and lived abroad in Paris and Belo Horizonte, Brazil, since leaving Ball State in 1994. Todd had been symptomatic for a couple of years by 1993, when my mom died, but he had never been seen by a neurologist. It was the mid–1990s when a genetic test for the SCAs began to be identified. I was unaware of this since nobody in my family saw a neurologist during this time.

Then Scott returned to Indiana after living in Brazil until 2005, clearly showing symptoms, and my dad took Scott to see a neurologist in Indianapolis. They would find out there was now an entire panel of tests which might tell him specifically what type our family had. Dad said that they were billed $2,500 for this test. When my dad confronted the doctor, unhappy about his not disclosing the cost, the doctor said he had no idea what the cost would be when he ordered it. This was not a genetic test that was requested at random or for exploratory purposes. This was a genetic panel of all 12 types of Ataxias that had been identified from 1993 to 2005. This genetic test would determine after more than 100 years of stabs in the dark what precise type of cerebellar degeneration had been wreaking havoc on our family.

Knowing he had SCA2 versus SCA6 did not help Scott live with his diagnosis. There were none then, and there would be no viable treatments for any of the SCAs in his lifetime. I never discussed this with Scott, but he had nothing to gain from being tested that I can see. But it did identify the type of SCA that Brian and I and then our cousins would utilize to find out if we had it. It also exposed a missing piece of the puzzle that I would use to help me construct our family's story. After Scott found out our family had SCA2, Brian was then tested in 2006. He tested negative for it and paid a much more reasonable cost for testing.

Brian went to Kokomo to visit cousins Jeff, Vickie, and Marti and told them that there was a blood test that could tell them if they were in fact positive for the family condition. Brian told them that it had been identified as SCA2, as Scott had found out. Since then they have all three tested negative so there will be no one affected by SCA2 in their family lines. Vickie has two children, two grandchildren and one great grandchild. Marti has two children and two grandchildren. My oldest brother Todd has never had a genetic test.

It was 2017, and although he wasn't driving anymore, Todd was occasionally joining my dad and brother Brian to go out to eat, go to the YMCA or to the grocery store. In the last year, he was noticeably doing less and going out less as it became increasingly difficult to transfer in out of his wheelchair. In his early 30s, Todd lived in Bloomington and was taking classes at IU. We actually ran into each other a couple times on campus while I was a freshman in Bloomington. He was living on the west side of town in a trailer and I was staying in the Foster-Harper dorm on campus. He also worked construction for Clifford, the contractor my dad used when he built his Nashville cabin in 1995. Working for Clifford involved climbing ladders to work on rooftops a few years after his symptoms began. After working for Clifford, he worked for a short time laying heavy stone until his employer told Todd that although he was a good worker, he could not afford the increased risk he posed due to his unsteadiness. When he was no longer able to do manual labor, he taught himself how to make dozens of chairs and tables, mostly from pine. Todd later bought a house in Bedford, Indiana, where he built a custom shed. He had always worked with his hands, as a mechanic just out of high school. Sean now owns the 1968 Porsche 912 Todd bought in 2000 that he used to drive and work on himself.

In early 2017 I was still working for CPM at Duke. For weeks, I had been contacting organizations whose job it was to assist the needs of people like Todd. My brother was now relying on a wheelchair and was living alone just down the road from my dad in Nashville, Indiana. My dad had just turned 77, and my older brother Brian, who consistently helped when needed, lived just over an hour away. It was time for other support to help navigate Todd's needs and assure that all the responsibility wasn't being placed on my dad.

I traveled back to Indiana in spring of 2017, this time to get our family together with Todd and his caseworker to decide what our next steps would be. When I arrived at the airport in Indianapolis, I rented a wheelchair accessible van and drove down to Nashville. I also wanted to give Todd the opportunity to go and do whatever he wanted without any barriers or constraints. Carol was one of many artists who was drawn to the beautiful and hilly area created by glaciers in southern Indiana. Carol and Todd dated initially and remained close friends for the next 25 years. Over the years, Todd and Carol had traveled to numerous sanctuaries in southern Indiana together. We had secretly been scheming for weeks to take Todd to the nearby Brown County State Park and the T.C. Steele Museum, where he used to work.

On Saturday Carol and I took Todd, who reluctantly agreed to join us, on an adventure in the van with an electronic ramp. He wanted to pick up groceries nearby in the newly opened Bean Blossom Dollar General. He was thrilled that the aisles were nice and wide and that we were nearly the only ones there shopping. Then we stopped by Carol's house in Nashville. She was remodeling her house. I jumped out and took a quick tour while Frankenstein the

Chihuahua mix hopped in the van with Todd. Next, we went to the Nashville Museum of Artifacts and he and Carol knew many of the local artists whose work was on display. Four hours later, we came home, and Todd was exhausted, and so were we.

We met with a social worker assigned to Todd by Thrive Alliance, a local organization that assisted people in local communities with the care they needed. We discussed as a family and with Todd what he needed and what our options were. She helped set in motion several different actions that helped ensure Todd was getting what he needed. And she helped us think about what we should consider for the future. Todd lived in a house less than a mile from my dad's house since the fall of 2004. He lived there with my brother Scott until his death in 2011 and lived there alone until the spring of 2018. He has been slowly progressing for over 25 years, longer than any of my grandfather Earl's descendants who were affected. We moved Todd out of his house and into a nursing home near my dad's in the spring of 2018.

HUMAN SPIRIT

I was down at Dad's cabin in Nashville, Indiana, chatting with him and his partner Peggy along with my brother Brian. In his usual fashion, Dad was describing in detail one of his many experiences from his childhood, living on the farm. Peggy said, "I can't remember those kinds of details in my past." My dad replied that he grew up hearing his father, Russell, telling stories constantly and usually about different people's connections to one another from the small, rural community in northern Indiana where he spent his entire life. Dad said it just came naturally for him to do this, like his father Russell had done.

Grandpa Creighton was a longtime member of the Gideons International, an evangelical Christian Association founded in 1899, and a trustee for the Haven Hubbard Home, a historic sanitarium in northern Indiana. In the early decades, this was part of a large working farm, complete with beef and dairy cows, hogs and poultry. Elderly residents were encouraged to help in the garden with chores and other duties. In addition, after a local community member died suddenly, Grandpa Creighton and my dad would help his widow and their daughter take care of their chickens. There are dozens of examples just like these about my grandpa.

I loved my grandpa and looked up to him with genuine admiration. Russell was a tall, strong, playful and a deeply caring human being. He was guided by his religion and he was helping people whenever he had an opportunity or could make one. Until that day talking with my dad, Peggy and Brian, I had never made an association between my own desire to establish connections with and between others that were ultimately centered on helping people. I think a combination of exposure to their ways and a heaping helping of neatly placed DNA is responsible for this characteristic in me.

My church in Durham had been a place I could go and be touched by either some part of the sermon, the music, or even a personal interaction with someone. This day I happened to be by myself and the service that day was led by two members, husband and wife. They gave a sermon titled "What Is Spirit?" and played the music as well, with Helen on the harp and Eric on guitar. I enjoyed the service thoroughly but got goosebumps when they spoke the closing words below.

Faith in God is optional, but faith in the self—in the **spirit** within, is imperative. Have faith in yourself. Have faith in the human first, then God if you want.

Abhijit Naskar

Go now in peace and let your spirit shine! Once we believe in ourselves, we can risk curiosity, wonder, spontaneous delight, or any experience that reveals the human spirit.

e.e. cummings

I was still in Toledo and this was after I had lost my mom. My grandpa Russell was in a nursing home in Warsaw and had his leg amputated below the knee after a lifetime of controlled diabetes was now out of control, at 92. He had not eaten in more than two weeks—he was well aware of what was happening to him: he was dying. I remember praying for God to "take him already," to ease his suffering. Atul Gawande wrote *Being Mortal* and reading this while I was writing helped me understand why I had felt so strongly about it.

> A landmark 2010 study from Massachusetts General Hospital had even more startling findings.... The result: those who saw a palliative care specialist stopped chemotherapy sooner, entered hospice care far earlier, experience less suffering at the end of their lives—*and they lived 25% longer*. In other words, our decision making in medicine has failed so spectacularly that we have reached the point of actively inflicting harm on patients rather than confronting the subject of mortality. If end of life discussions were an experimental drug, the FDA would approve it [177].

Facing our mortality is something we try not to think about. Although it was indirectly, I dipped my toes into exploring what I wanted to pass on to my daughter. This was written in 2016 while I was participating in an expressive writing course and without making a direct connection to how it was intertwined to my purpose in life.

> Kendall,
>
> I wish you a life full of happiness and joy that I see in your eyes every day. You have such a gift for expressing yourself and seeing your joy always lifts my spirits. There may be a time when you struggle with what life may bring and when that time comes please focus on what you are grateful for and never forget the joy you create by just being present and engaged. You have blessed my life in a way you may not ever understand. You have given to me such a strong sense of purpose to continue to excel and never be satisfied. The joy I see when you are fully engaged in anything, playing, singing, dancing, gives me so much happiness. Please don't ever forget this joy and remember that we are both so lucky to have found each other.

Kendall does not know much of her birth mother's story, but she will know exactly how she fits into mine. She was a piece of my own spirit that I found on the day she was born and stronger than any strand of DNA could ever be. Our spirit is something that I had been totally underestimating my whole life. Since I have been writing for almost three years now, I have been connecting to family, some of whom are deceased and I had never met. I knew my mother and brother Scott well—connecting to their spirit was not only cathartic but was imperative for me to write my story.

I still had more to learn about the human spirit. Liz and I shared a special connection and had been just acquaintances then casual friends while our children aged through preschool together in Chapel Hill. Right when I was separating from Sean, we became much closer friends. My connection to Liz also extended from her mom to me. Mercedes offered to let Kendall and me stay in her Brooklyn apartment while we toured New York City in the summer of 2014. It was a fantastic trip and I introduced Kendall to everything the city had to offer in one week—Central Park, the Hall of Science, a mini musical performance in Bryant Park. The *Bullets Over Broadway* performance of "I've Got a New Baby" that was sung that day by Zach Braff and Betsy Wolfe is one that I still swoon over to this day.

Mercedes traveled from Brooklyn to Chapel Hill for Thanksgiving in 2016, where I hosted a potluck dinner. Liz and I along with our four kids now functioned more like family than just friends. The weather was mild, and we sat outside after eating and enjoyed the weather and conversation. A week later, I answered the phone early in the morning and it was Liz's sister, Jasmine, in New York. She told me she had not been able to contact Liz all night, and since I lived near her, she asked if I could get a message to her to call her sister. Jasmine did not say anything else, but I knew what happened from the sound of her voice. Liz was in massage therapy school and was helping my neighbor three houses down with his three school-aged girls a couple days a week in the morning. As soon as I got off the phone, I drove down to see if she was there. She was—I caught her as she was about to enter the front door. I told her she needed to call Jasmine right away and offered her my phone. I think she sensed the urgency, and I just grabbed her and held her tight. I told her I would get the girls to school and she went home to call her sister.

Mercedes had passed away suddenly on December 4, 2016, at 62. The funeral was in Brooklyn that next Thursday, and although I had not talked to Liz about going, I needed to be there. After flying to New Jersey, taking a train to the city, the metro to Brooklyn, and a cab to the funeral home, I walked in well into the service. A family friend was singing "You Are So Beautiful," which immediately overwhelmed me with emotion. Her pastor then told stories about Mercedes and how she cared deeply for her family and friends which was visibly evident to everyone. I could literally feel her spirit come alive as I felt the entire room giving thanks for her life.

I picked up an Amanda Palmer book in the airport in Newark, never having heard of her before. I devoured this book on the trip home from Mercedes' funeral. In November 2014, Palmer released her memoir *The Art of Asking*, which expands on a TED Talk she gave. I loved Amanda's descriptions of making powerful and meaningful connections with others, usually strangers. After she graduated from college she would dress in all white and stand perched on a crate, *The Eight Foot Bride*, in Harvard Square, Cambridge. She would stand there perfectly still until a bystander would drop some money in a hat and then she would look into their eyes and "thank" them by handing them a single flower. Years later, she would follow the same principle when she began asking the fans of her band The Dresden Dolls to help her raise money. She gathered $1.2 million on her first crowdsourcing attempt. This feat was not based on her business acumen but on her pure understanding of human connection.

I was a big proponent of the benefits that human connection can provide, including massage. My dad took me to my first massage when I was in high school. I had gone every few months for at least five years. My current go-to massage therapist was Ryan. Coincidently, our friendship would have a dramatic impact on me. It was 2012, I had recently separated from Sean and he had our daughter for the night. I was already in a highly emotional state, and Ryan was everything that I needed that day. He was a smoking hot, tattooed, motorcycle riding masseuse with a Zen-like nature and a calming presence. He responded to my chaotic exterior with loving understanding. I remember he said I was like a delicate flower that day, which was true then but hopefully will not be ever again.

He happened to also be a bartender at a local restaurant, so I would occasionally drop in to eat and we would talk. We maintained a purely platonic friendship. He gave me so much. That first year we knew each other, he shared with me that he lost his brother to suicide. And we bonded over a spiritual moment that he shared about his brother that demonstrated to me that someone's spirit can live long after they're physically gone. He had recently left the spa I went to, so I thought I would try a facial to mix it up.

Danielle was a new aesthetician at the salon, and when we met, we had an instant affection and appreciation for each other. She was tall and beautiful and she had an ethereal quality that was deeply comforting to me. She started my facial and asked me if I had ever tried high frequency. I replied no. She explained that it was a wand powered by an electric frequency that is used to clear and smooth out your complexion. I told her to give it a try. Within the first five minutes I felt my right lower leg jump! I didn't say a word, and even played it off, like you would if you accidentally fell asleep in class. Even afterward, I played it off to myself as a coincidence and a fluke.

After a day or two I noticed a calm and increased balance that I didn't at first even contribute to anything. Then I Googled high frequency facials to find out how they work. Two different things may have been going on. The first was that the different frequency of energy used to help my facial complexion was also affecting my neurotransmitters linked to my ongoing depression. The other was that the frequency waves had traveled down my neuropathways in my body, and when they reached my right lower leg, the jolt I felt was when it bridged a literal gap in the neural connection.

A few weeks later, I scheduled another facial and I told Danielle what my experience had been like. We discussed what might have taken place that day, including that maybe it signified absolutely nothing—nothing except that there was in fact hope that there were several possibilities with alternative therapies that are not "mainstream." Danielle mentioned that she was certified in Reiki. I had a very general knowledge of what it was, but it really was a mystery to me. I did know that Danielle was by far the most spiritual presence I had ever met, and if I was ever going to try Reiki, it would be with her.

Having Reiki done for the first time was a wonderful experience. To feel someone directing their positive energy toward me was exhilarating. After an hour-long session, we exchanged words for the first time. We independently spoke about a connection with a shared energy that was continuously in motion back and forth, as if we were communicating the entire time. It made me think I must try to carve out time for this, where my thoughts were being driven by something other than conscious ones.

WRITE TO HEAL

I stumbled upon another transformative experience although this one depended on a steady flow of conscious and subconscious thoughts. Putting down on paper my own perspective of what had happened to me was beneficial. This was necessary to know how and why I had made decisions throughout my life that were all connected to my family's story. And my story was initially not "told" to anyone—it was a chance to retell the story to myself. In April 2015 I had been working at Duke for seven years as a research coordinator and I was on the Duke Integrative Medicine listserv. A research study was being advertised to get research subjects to participate. The cost for enrolling in the six-week workshop was nearly $400 but participating in the research study was free. To me, free services were as good as monetary compensation. Elizabeth, whom I knew from working with her on the health coaching project a few years prior, was the research coordinator for this study. I immediately called her and signed up.

I had never heard of using expressive writing to help process traumatic events, but I was game for just about anything—especially since it was different than anything I had already tried and it was free. The classes were held on Saturday mornings from 10 until 12 for six weeks, which was perfect for me. I went into the first class without high expectations of what may come out of it. I skipped the "suggested reading" about how this class was designed to work. But I did show up faithfully each Saturday and spill my guts to a lined composition notebook. Here is the original advertisement to recruit research subjects.

Transform Your Health: Write to Heal

This workshop is designed to help you discover ways to manage stressful events and upheavals in your life through writing. The act of writing engages internal healing resources that affect mental and physical health. Expressive writing has the power to help you reduce heart rate and blood pressure, minimize stress, strengthen the immune system, and improve your self-esteem.

Transform Your Health: Write to Heal is a transformative six-week workshop that helps you access your inner healing voice. You do not need to have writing experience or aspirations to participate. The instructor will lead you through a progression of restorative ranking exercises. The workshop employs different modes of writing that help you deal in unique ways including:

Expressive writing, which removes obstacles and moves you beyond a personal, private emotional upheaval or crisis.

Transactional writing, which allows you to take care of unfinished business conveys your feelings, expectations, and intentions for yourself and others, ingratitude, compassion, forgiveness and lovingkindness.

Poetic writing, which uses narrative structure and metaphor to tell your story as you wish to tell.

Affirmative writing, which centers work focus on your best qualities and how you would like to express your life in the future.

Legacy writing, which teaches you to write others about your values, major life lessons, turning points and epiphanies.

The prompts were provided in a structured way, so we all knew what the others were writing about, but we didn't see each other's work. After each writing prompt was given, I responded by filling in my own notebook with my writing. No one except me looked at, read or analyzed what I wrote in my journal. On one particular Saturday, I did not feel the need to respond to "tell a story about your list of strengths." I wrote in my journal, "I am not feeling this, and I can't think of a story." At that time in my life, I was not able to see the forest for the trees. I had written an entire page of my strengths, yet I did not feel capable of telling a story based on them. I didn't know what my story could be yet. Here is a description of what expressive writing is.

> Expressive writing literally comes from our core. It is personal and emotional writing without regard to form or other writing conventions, like spelling, punctuation, and verb agreement. Turn off your resident Dr. Comma Splice. Expressive writing pays no attention to propriety: it simply expresses what is on your mind and in your heart [Evans, *Write Yourself Well*].

I would attend the scheduled class each week and sit in the front of the class. Without fail, especially in the first few weeks, I would have tears streaming down my face as I wrote. It was painful to write about the experiences, but I also found that writing evoked deep emotions that were different from simply recalling events in my mind and talking about them. Writing about traumatic events allowed me space to put my story in my own terms and edit my story the way that I wanted it to be framed.

The series of writing exercises that I wrote in my notebook back in 2016 would help me begin the very rough first draft of this book. It never occurred to me during the six-week course that this was anything other than a productive mental exercise. Part of the brilliance of the expressive writing class was how it was structured: writing about traumatic experiences at the beginning and mindful and affirmative writing at the end. The writing was the key that opened the door of my soul to be able to explore all the many factors at play throughout my life, including what my purpose was.

Writing about my innermost feelings was a way for me to heal, mostly from what I had gone through emotionally, not just the trauma caused by the condition's effect on members of my family, but also the silence and secrecy surrounding their life and death. The process of writing about the trauma was quelled by the fact that I didn't have to bring anyone else up to speed. My thoughts were a one-way street, and no one was questioning me about what, why or how something happened. I had successfully lived more than four decades without being able to articulate exactly what my life had been like living in a family affected by cerebellar degeneration or Ataxia, not to myself and surely not to anyone else.

I had seen a handful of therapists since 2007 with varying degrees of success. I cannot count the number of therapy sessions during which I was trying to explain what happened throughout my life and how I felt about it. It did not matter how I felt about it happening to me. It mattered that the story that I told myself was meaningful to me in a way that it could never be to someone else. My neurologist referred me to an excellent therapist in late 2014. She had experience leading a support group for families affected by Huntington's Disease, which shares similarities with Ataxia, so she understood some of my worries and fears, but she retired six months after I found her. I'm sure many of my therapists would have done anything to have me relax and just talk. I wanted to, but I didn't have the words to explain what had happened to me. This was the very first prompt I responded to on the first day of the class.

2016—Transform Your Health writing prompt: "most traumatic experience of your life"

The death of my mother shook me to the core because it was sudden, shocking, and deliberate. A deliberate choice on her part to end her life, end her marriage, and for me an end of ever having a mother again. It still brings me to tears to relive this event—the thought of this loss, my father having to find her body and having to see my brother's reactions to their irreversible loss. It was a permanent loss, but we had emotionally lost her years before.

From the time she was diagnosed, after years of different doctors telling her she was fine. Watching her unable to hold in her anger and frustration and hearing her moaning and crying, pleading for someone to hear her calls for help from her bedroom at night. The pain she felt seemed to damage her ability to accept and give love.

I think she felt that withholding her love would make her life and other's lives less painful. This proved to have certainly made it more pain-filled for everyone. I was angry at her for doing this to my dad, my brothers and me. How dare she cause so much pain in the last years of her life and then take her own.

> Anger, shame, guilt, humiliation,
> shame, anger, fear
> fear, anger, shame.

After writing my own narrative the words "anger, shame, guilt, humiliation" and so on spilled out of me. These words were never said to me by my mom, but she didn't need to say them to communicate these feelings to me. In the same way I knew she loved me I knew this too. My mom was not able to verbalize her pain because she was so ashamed of what and how it all happened. More than a year after writing this down in my notebook I ran across Brené Brown's explanation of guilt versus shame, which made almost perfect sense to me, in her book *Daring Greatly*.

> In fact, as we work to understand shame, one of the simpler reasons that shame is so difficult to talk about is vocabulary. We often use the terms embarrassment, guilt, humiliation and shame interchangeably. It might seem overly picky to stress the importance of using the appropriate term to describe an experience or emotion; however, it is much more than semantics.
>
> How we experience these different emotions comes down to self-talk. How do we talk to ourselves about what is happening? The best place to start examining self-talk and untangling these four distinct emotions is with shame and guilt. The majority of shame researchers and clinicians agree is best understood as the difference between "I am bad" and "I did something bad."
>
> Guilt=I did something bad
> Shame=I am bad [71]

A few weeks after completing the course Transform Your Health: Write to Heal, I wanted to share with my dad what appeared to be so helpful to me, so I sent him this email.

> Dad,
>
> I would attend the scheduled class each week and sit in the front of the class. Without fail, especially in the first 3–4 weeks I would have tears streaming down my face as I wrote. It was painful to write about the

experiences, but I also found that writing evoked deep emotions that were different from simply recalling events in my mind and talking about them. Writing about traumatic events allowed me space to put my story in my own terms and edit my story the way that I wanted it to be framed.

Dana

From: Bob Creighton
Sent: Wednesday, April 27, 2016 4:10 p.m.
To: Dana Creighton
Subject: Re: Expressive Writing Class

I'm glad you did this class. It seems like it has helped somewhat even though there's nothing that will erase the bulk of the emotional pain.

I love you very much and will do whatever I can to help.

Love, Dad

My dad knew firsthand that the emotional pain I had been carrying around could never be "erased." I knew this too, but I had found a way that I could write my version of the same story that ended so tragically. Almost a year after undergoing the writing project, I came to understand that my entire life experience had aligned itself such that there was no other way than for me to tell my story. I reached a point that I needed to share a seemingly tragic set of circumstances that have been reframed. I realized that it might be possible to tell my story in a way that others could follow.

It was not reasonable to believe that one type of therapy alone would temper the emotional pain I was dealing with. I chose to adopt as many as I could that could potentially help me. I was open to alternative therapies and my experience was overwhelmingly positive. I appreciated the systematic and simple approach to writing. The structured setting of the classroom made it easy for me to set aside the time and follow the writing prompts. The prompts were simple and structured logically. Compared to traditional therapy sessions I had in the past, I enjoyed the freedom to follow the path of my own thoughts. I also liked the flexibility to switch trains of thought based on self-directed thoughts and feelings. Writing about traumatic events in my past allowed me to express myself in a way that gave me a sense of acceptance and peace about my life that I had not found before.

Maya Angelou said, "There is no greater sorrow than bearing an untold story inside you," and now I completely understand why. My story reframed has given me a sense of calm and clarity about my past, a clarity that I never imagined existed as well as a renewed hope for the future. And by sharing my story, I want to encourage others to seek their own truth by recognizing what their own experiences can reveal about what is present but may not be apparent. I also realized how important it may be for others in similar circumstances to know what we share. I needed to tell this story for others who have undergone trauma but were not capable of expressing their pain or of making sense of the remnants. I had successfully lived more than four decades without being able to articulate exactly what my life had been like living in a family affected by Ataxia, not to myself and surely not to anyone else. To acknowledge the pain I was feeling and to attempt to understand where it was coming from was an insurmountable task to me. I was so afraid of giving into powerful emotions that threatened to sink my ship that I had painstakingly and slowly built over the past 30 years. I tried desperately to portray myself to others as if nothing was wrong.

The end result of the participants' writing was not why the study was being done. I did, however, complete a *post-writing reflections* form with my feedback about how I felt about each writing prompt and what it felt like to express my feelings in this specific way. Our personal responses to how different prompts felt to us were unique. This was the data that was gathered for this study, along with the depression scales that were completed before classes began on the first day and then again on the last day of class, six weeks apart. At the completion of class, I was glad I did this and just continued on, not thinking much more about it. This intensive writing experience was cathartic—expressing my perceptions and realizations in a way I had never done before.

One of the many ways that the writing experience was so powerful for me was going through the process of granting forgiveness.

It was a way that I could take my mind to a place that I had physically not been yet or would never be able to go. This was taken from one of the legacy writing prompts written around week four of the six-week course.

2016 Expressive Writing Course prompt: letter to Mom "granting forgiveness letter"

Mom,

I have forgiven you for both ending your own life and for withholding your personal emotions with me. I understand that it would have been too painful for you to share your feelings of fear, anger and guilt with me. And I would never have understood or granted you the right to do what you did.

I forgive you also for sharing certain fears with me—telling me I was never going to be able to have a baby—this was selfish, and yet, I forgive you. I find it incredibly difficult to express my emotions about this and the pain that I had throughout my entire childhood.

I choose to take those experiences I had and turn them into useful lessons. I want to be able to have gone through them and still have the ability to wholeheartedly love people in my life. I chose a plan that no one can choose for me. Only I can decide who I am and how I love. I pray my daughter never has to go through the pain I felt when you were ill and ... then gone forever.

Dana

What appeared on paper in front of me were my very thoughts explained in a way that made more sense to me than the circumstances surrounding them ever could. The process of writing had a profound but surreptitious impact on me. After finishing the writing course, I tucked my journal away in my closet and closed the door. Several weeks later I ran into John Evans, the instructor of the course. We were both waiting for our children's group tennis lesson to finish. We chatted a little about the writing study and he told me he was also a health coach. I didn't pull this notebook back out of my closet until weeks into meeting with John as my health coach.

Chapter VI

Love Is the Law

Love is the law. Love is not ruled by laws.
All is enough. There is no higher call.
Every light shines from a single flame.
You Shall Love in Heaven's name.
All is enough. There is no higher call.
　　　　　　　　　　　—Jonathan Byrd

The Power of Your Mind

Starting to write led to focusing on mindfulness which led to writing a memoir. One of the benefits I reaped from this progression of events was having an increased and a highly functioning sense of intuition. I had been frequenting Patina, a consignment store for home furniture in Durham. I had been there several times in the last few weeks mostly to window shop. One of those afternoons, a local jewelry maker, Sherry, was selling her necklaces there. Among the many things in the store I was fond of were her big beaded necklaces with large metal crosses. Though there were a variety of colors, blue, green, and white, the coral color really stood out in my mind as stunning. As had happened many times before, I left that day without buying anything.

Several weeks later I was picking up the chair that I purchased at a thrift store and had repainted at Patina. I really wanted one of those necklaces and they weren't in the store anymore. I asked the owner for Sherry's contact information. Another few weeks went by and her phone number went from my purse to the kitchen table where it sat some more. Then, on Saturday July 22, 2017, my longtime friend from childhood called to tell me my uncle Dave, my dad's younger brother, had died suddenly in his sleep at 74. Dave was the baby in my dad's family. Dave's youngest son Brandon was two years older than me and he had always been a good friend as well as a cousin. Kendall and I had just stayed at Brandon's house and spent the week in Warsaw right before his father's death. We had spent a lot of time with Dave and Mary Anne, his wife of 36 years. We had shared meals and often swam in the pool at their house during the day as Dave prepared the outside area for a family get-together that night. Kendall and I enjoyed the family reunion that Sunday with 129 family members showing up. That summer visit to my annual family reunion had not happened since Kendall was a toddler.

On that Sunday after hearing the news of Dave's passing, I booked a flight to go back to Indiana, again, on Tuesday for his funeral on Wednesday. On Monday morning, the day before I left for Indiana, something inside me made me need to call Sherry and tell her that I needed to buy one of her necklaces and, if possible, that day. She said, "Absolutely," and she gave me her address. I picked out my necklace with oversized beads and a large metal cross that I wore to my uncle Dave's funeral. I can only describe my sudden need to have that necklace as a way I could pay tribute to his undying spirit.

The day before I flew to Warsaw to attend my uncle's funeral, I called Jamel to see if I could stop by his house. He had introduced me to many ideas and books that fascinated me, and we often discussed the power of one's mind or spirituality. I wanted to borrow the book *The Power of Your Subconscious Mind* by Dr. Joseph Murphy, published in 1963. At his house, back in 2013, I had only read parts of this book. I was now driven by a need to read it in its entirety. I couldn't find it anywhere online, because I didn't remember the exact title. I had bugged him several times over the last few weeks that I wanted to borrow it, so the day before my flight he was home, and I stopped by his house and got it, thankfully. I was reading this book from cover to cover this time around.

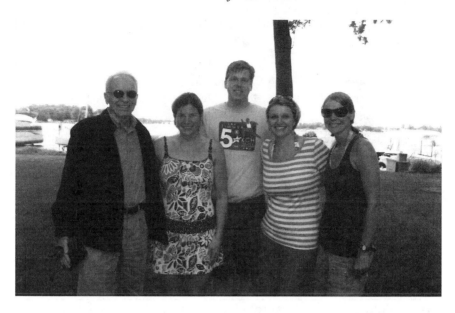

(From left) Robert Creighton, Angie Hartley, Brandon Creighton, Dana Creighton and Liza Arnold at a summer vacation visit to Winona Lake, Indiana, 2010.

While I was in Warsaw for my uncle's funeral, I stayed with Angie and her family. Angie was a lifelong friend who had been my basketball teammate from fourth grade through high school.

She and my brother Scott were in the same grade, one year ahead of me. Angie was the childhood friend who called me to tell me about my uncle's death that Saturday morning while I was watching Kendall's horseback riding lesson. As I sit down and read this book on her porch, I was struck when I read these words.

> Let the words of my mouth...
> ***(your thoughts, mental images)***
> and the meditation of my heart...
> ***(your feelings, nature, emotion)***
> be acceptable in thy sight O Lord...
> ***(the law of your subconscious mind)***
> my strength and my redeemer.
> ***(the power and wisdom of your subconscious mind that
>   can redeem you from sickness, bondage, and misery)***
> [Psalms 19:14, *The Power of Your Subconscious Mind* 111].

I must have read this at least a dozen times trying to figure out why it was eerily familiar.

> Let the words of my mouth and the meditation of my heart be acceptable in thy sight O Lord, my strength and my redeemer [Psalms 19:14].

It didn't come to me right away, but as I took a break from reading on her screened-in porch and just let those words sink into my mind, I realized that as a teenager I used to recite that verse each and every time before I would pray.

LOSING MY RELIGION

From the time I was young, we all attended church as a family. As I got older, I thought of religion as a necessary ritual, like attending school. I didn't necessarily love school or church, but gave each one my full attention when it was required. The values and lessons learned while attending church functions were vital to shaping who I was as a human being. I thoroughly enjoyed the social aspect and fellowship that came with church. As competing priorities sprang up, I embraced them, but continued to live according to my beliefs learned in church. I was consistent and kept up daily prayers by giving thanks for my many blessings. I don't remember specifically praying for certain things or outcomes. I focused on acknowledging what I had to be grateful for.

When we brought Kendall home at eight days old, both Sean's mom and my dad came to help us for several days. Sean affectionately appointed my dad as Kendall's "Papa C." She was our only child and his only grandchild. I have and will try my best to pass on the valuable lessons I learned at a young age to my daughter. She already has a head start since my dad has been writing her letters several times a year since she could read. Papa C and Kendall share a special bond, but they don't get to see each other more than a few times a year. He has written to her about the meaning and relevance of words like ability, acceptance and attitude. Around Christmas last year he wrote about how not all religions celebrate the same things and how they often think differently about many different subjects.

I took a religion class that I thoroughly enjoyed as a freshman at Indiana University. We studied and read about many different theologies, and it was because of this class that the summer after my mom died I read *When Bad Things Happen to Good People* by Harold Kushner. He described the circumstances of his seemingly healthy baby who was diagnosed with progeria at two and died at 14. He explained how this tragedy led him to question his beliefs in the Jewish traditions he had been trained in as a rabbi and consider how religion and God can help us to overcome our pain and sorrow. It was a window into a different version of religion that seemed to make sense to me and was at the same time comforting.

After my mom died, I continued to pray, perhaps less than wholeheartedly. Eventually, it just did not make sense for me to give thanks for the pain and emptiness I was left with. I took about a 14-year hiatus from conventional religion. When Kendall came along, I wanted to give her a chance to belong somewhere she could have experiences like I had. It was just the two of us, even though this was only two years into the marriage. Sean had been working the night shift at the burn center at UNC on and off for years. He was typically coming home from the night shift at the hospital and he would sleep on Sunday mornings. I searched for and tried out several nondenominational churches in Chapel Hill and Durham. I landed at Eno River Unitarian Universalist Fellowship (ERUUF), just down the road from us in Durham. I loved everything about it—the sanctuary with the view of the woods, the preacher, her sermons and the fantastic music. ERUUF is inclusive of different theologies; many pagans are members.

> *The mission of the Eno River Unitarian Universalist Fellowship is to transform lives by building a free and inclusive covenantal religious community of spirit, service, justice, and love.*

I was far from a regular, but in addition to attending services I would try out different church-affiliated events and groups a few times a year. I listened to speakers and attended small group sessions. I watched then discussed documentaries like *I Am Not Your Negro* about James Baldwin and *Being Mortal* with Atul Gawande. I attended Death Café, where we discussed our own mortality and why it was important to talk about it, facilitated by the church's leader of pastoral care. When I would decide to be present, I found that it would add insight to subjects that were important to me. The more I gave the more I received what I needed.

When I was in the middle of writing my story, I went to get a coffee at a nearby bookstore. I ordered a cappuccino with hazelnut like Scott used to drink. After he introduced me to it at a bookstore in Bloomington, Indiana, I started drinking it too. I quickly gave in to my urge to peruse the biography section just next to the café. I stumbled upon the book *Wild*. I saw it for the first time at the end of the aisle, but I passed it by among the others it was grouped with. Then I headed down the other side of the aisle and ran across it again. It stuck out for me because on the cover was a lone old-school, brown hiking boot with red shoestrings, just like my brother Scott used to wear.

The title and author were vaguely familiar, and I paused. I had read about this book in another memoir. At this point I bought it, knowing I needed to find out what the author's story was. After her mother's death when Cheryl Strayed was 22, she thought she had lost everything. Her family had scattered, and her own marriage was soon destroyed. With no experience or training, she hiked more than a thousand miles on the Pacific Crest Trail (PCT)—alone. Its corridor through the United States is in California, Oregon, and Washington. I raced through this book as I felt such a connection to her story.

> I prayed and prayed, then faltered. Not because I couldn't find God, because suddenly I absolutely did: God was there, I realized, and God had no intention of making things happen or not, saving my mother's life. God is not a granter of wishes. God was a ruthless bitch [23].

I never would have admitted this, but this was exactly how I felt after I lost my mom. I had never thought about my giving up on prayer as giving up on God completely. I still had a waning faith, but I just wasn't going to act like I was grateful when I really wasn't. The year my mom died, I struggled both in my classes and in basketball. My heart was not with either one. I was incredibly private, keeping all my feelings to myself. My junior and senior years were comparatively much better. Both years I was consistent and hardworking on the defensive end, as my team was never lacking for points. I was a co-captain on my senior team, and we made a strong run in the NCAA tournament, losing to Old Dominion on their home court in the second round.

I was honestly relieved that my basketball career had come to an end.

Bridging the Gap

After my mom died, while I had lost my desire to follow religion as I had previously, I bridged the gap in my faith through music. This really had emerged as being a part of my story until I was writing so much that it finally rose to the surface. In May 2017 I was attending ERUUF, *"How will you use your gift? It can be hardest to see the light flashing in front of us."* Beloved Community Chorus was performing at church as part of the service that day. They sang "Heaven Help Us All" originally sung by Stevie Wonder in 1970. I couldn't believe this was the first time I had ever heard this song. I went home and looked up his version and I was compelled to listen to it over and over. This song exemplifies that everyone has their own unique struggle. But we can garner hope that someone may offer us some help. Some are born into and are raised with religion as a tool to help defend against what life can hand us.

This would be a strong asset for Martin Luther King, Jr., during his lifetime, along with his gift of being able to see a vision of this world that not many people could see and having the skills of a master communicator. When *Selma* came out in theaters, I went and saw it by myself. I was born in 1973 and grew up in a small town of mostly whites in northern Indiana. I of course was familiar with the history of Martin Luther King, Jr., but I wanted to get a better picture of how the actual events in history developed and played out. This was as close as I could get to seeing how these events unfolded as I was not there to see them in real time.

Watching and deeply connecting with his and black people's struggles that occurred over three months in 1965 in Alabama had a much more dramatic and visceral impact than I could ever have imagined. I was amazed by the incredible journey this man led.

As the credits rolled down the screen I was overcome by strong emotions as I stayed in my seat and let my tears stream down my face. While I thought Kendall was too young to see the movie, I showed her the video of John Legend and Common's song "Glory." We talked about what had happened then and what the song represented.

I was also touched by other songs that were focused on fighting for freedom or justice. In 2003, I stumbled upon Rhiannon Giddens while she was playing with the Carolina Chocolate Drops at the Shakori Hills Music Festival about 25 miles from Chapel Hill. She is a native of Greensboro, North Carolina, and she was the lone female, one of three who played old-time country music with the fiddle and banjo. Their music was truly different than mainstream, and I loved it. I followed them for several years and when Rhiannon went solo, I was a fan of her unique sound and incredible voice. Her songs as a solo artist were a musical transformation of stories from history.

> Know thy history. Let it horrify you; let it inspire you. Let it show you how the future can look, for nothing in this world has not come around before. These songs are based on slave narratives from the 1800s, African American experiences of the last century, and the Civil Rights movement of the 1960s and headlines from streets of Ferguson and Baltimore today. Voices demanding to be heard, to impart the hard-earned wisdom of a tangled, difficult, complicated history; we just try to open the door and let them through [Giddens, *Freedom Highway*].

On *Freedom Highway*, Rhiannon tells this story that was inspired by the young girl whose owner had written an advertisement for her sale. She was "young and strong" and her nine-month old baby was "at the purchaser's option." Listening to this story that she envisioned belonged to this young human being whose sale was being treated as anything but human was very moving. I saw her in concert in Raleigh's Memorial Hall in 2018 and introduced Kendall to her artistic creativity and soulful presence.

I am a fan of Katy Perry and Kendall was an even bigger one. On her own, she decided to dress as the singer for Halloween when she was three years old. The following year, my friend Liz introduced us to KIDS BOP music CDs, the watered-down renditions of popular songs that she had gotten for her daughter Iliana, who was three years older than Kendall. The kids loved hearing all the popular songs sung by kids themselves. Four years later we had accumulated at least eight different CDs. Rather than searching on the radio for music, she would often just have me put in her latest favorite.

"Rise" was sung by a KIDZ BOP artist and was on the latest and greatest. When I first heard it, I didn't pay attention or listen to the words. I would hear this song day after day after day. Eventually I was hooked on it and I would go to YouTube and watch the video by Katy Perry. The lyrics spoke to me and for weeks I didn't even realize why I had connected so intensely. After starting this book, I wrote down the songs I had a deep connection to. After looking at each of the lyrics, I was astounded at the similarities they shared. Again, this song was centered on fighting back against continuous hurdles.

Since I've been writing for the past three years, I have been nostalgically listening to music. I was in the front row when I saw American legend John Mellencamp with Carlene Carter perform in his *Sad Clowns & Hillbillies* tour. Julie and I almost got to see Loretta Lynn in Durham but she suffered a stroke the day the concert was scheduled. I would often revisit many of the artists I have talked about in this book on my computer or on Pandora. Delta Rae will always be the group that I connect with the most.

When she was two, I took Kendall to Southpoint Mall in Durham to a free outdoor concert. Delta Rae was a local band, just starting out. After the concert they were handing out free CDs, so I took one. I really liked their music and it was no surprise that Kendall danced to the live music the entire night. A few days later, we took a shopping trip to the outlet mall in Smithfield. The CD had only five songs on it, but I played it repeatedly the entire trip, coming and going. Kendall couldn't even talk yet, but on the way home she had memorized the songs enough to "sing" along and she mimicked the harmonies and chorus as if she knew them.

My daughter and I discovered Delta Rae together in Durham in 2010, and within the next five years, I saw them live twice, once with Kendall at an outdoor festival in Raleigh and once by myself at the Cat's Cradle in Carrboro. I would typically listen to the songs that I was familiar with. I had seen some publicity about "No Peace in Quiet," a more recent song I had never heard. It was written about lead singer Ian's gut-wrenching breakup. He spoke about how painful the quiet moments in his life were, a constant reminder of what he had lost, and how he used that pain to summon the courage to move to Nashville like he had always wanted to do. I cried when I heard the words sung by his bandmate Liz.

I felt a similar pain my whole life when, inside, I was begging to figure out why and all I heard was silence. In 2016, I filled a notebook of my thoughts and feelings about my life and I began talking to John about it on a regular basis. This process had triggered something in me that I couldn't deny, and I reached out to someone different who could help me fill in the information I needed. I had been reaching out to people my whole life, but without identifying any specific intentions, I would come up short.

It was the fall of 2017 and my health coach, now my writing coach, and I were barely able to keep up with all the information I had been accumulating through my own research as well as the other connections I was continually making. We would routinely go over our allotted one-hour weekly session. Among the many suggestions that John would propose to me was to practice rowing. Over time I decided to give it a go. Using the ergometer was to me mind-numbing and counter-productive to my exercise routine. Then

I decided to get a rowing coach to help me someday learn to row on the water. What is the point of pretending to do something on a machine that could be done for real? I was like a nerd on tech day as I learned the proper form for each leg of the stroke. My coach eventually acquired a handmade rowing simulator built by her dad in his basement. It had actual oars that mimicked the experience of being on the water, requiring me to practice the rowing strokes efficiently to remain on the machine with steadiness.

Two years later John asked me out of the blue if I wanted to take a ride on the water. I hadn't been practicing at all at this point—not even on an ergometer. He said, "what if you take a ride with me and my coach?" "Hell yes!" I said. The following Saturday we met at Jordan Lake at 6 a.m. and prepared the 20-year-old, custom-made, three-person shell for the water. After Dan, the most experienced rower, got in, John helped my wobbly self into the middle position. Then John inserted himself and we pushed off into the dark with John leading us. Just like in my life, John was leading me into the dark not knowing what I was going to wander into. Roughly an hour into our ride we turned around and headed back. The sun was shining brightly, and we could now see and feel the sun and its warmth that was behind us all along.

CONNECTIONS

I was in high gear writing my story as well as reading books non-stop. It would prove to be like using watercolors, as I wouldn't know exactly what the figure on the page was until it appeared directly in front of me. I used a combination of single-digit typing and a voice recognition program. As the story continued to take shape, I was inundated with unexpected connections related to events that happened throughout my entire life. For instance, in 2003, after giving blood at the annual UNC campus Red Cross blood drive, I was waiting for my co-worker Barb to finish. I was walking around the Dean E. Smith Center, the "Dean Dome," looking at pictures. I didn't mind waiting; it was my first time in the legendary building. When she finished, we proceeded down the very long staircase outside to return to work. It was raining, and I had an umbrella in one hand, my planner in the other. My heel slipped off one of the first few steps. I fell directly on my ass with both hands holding onto something, not available to break my fall, almost like when I was four with a hockey stick and didn't have my hands available to break my fall in our basement.

I promptly passed out from the shock of the hard plunge to the concrete steps. I ended up in the ER, but this time luckily my backside took the brunt of the fall and not my head. What I experienced when I passed out was incredibly scary—I was desperately trying, but I was not able to form any thoughts. I was in a black hole–like experience where things were swirling around like a tornado, but nothing was identifiable, no words, no pictures. It was a chaos that I had never before or have since experienced. It was so surreal that I guess I stopped trying to make sense out of it. Years later, after reading more, I came to the realization that it may have been my subconscious thoughts and events that I had not yet processed at that time. I had the information and events stored in my brain which were numerous throughout my life, and when I passed out and then came to, they leapt headfirst into my consciousness, not knowing they were not welcomed.

For years, I was unable to effectively communicate this experience. When I attempted to recreate this event to John, I used similar language to how I described it above. Once again, talking through mechanisms of what might have happened gave me the words to explain it.

I was reading a book by Mark Wolynn weeks after I had written the section above. I read the following explanation of non-declarative memories and was shocked to realize the parallels to what might have occurred in my experience.

> Traumatic experiences are often stored as non-declarative memory. When an event becomes so overwhelming that we lose our words, we cannot accurately record or "declare" the memory in story form,

which requires language to do so. It's as though a flash flood is streaming through all doors and windows at once. In the danger we don't stop
long enough to put our experience into words. We just leave the house.
    Without words we no longer have full access to our memory of the
event. Fragments of experience go unnamed and submerged out of
sight. Lost and undeclared, they become part of our unconscious [*It
Didn't Start with You* 55].

I read this description about not having the words to explain our
perspective limits our ability to communicate to ourselves or anyone else. I could relate to this so closely and I could also feel how
other family members likely struggled with this. In 2006, I was still
at UNC but in a new position and with a different department. This
position was cut only a year after I was hired. I was on unemploy-
ment for several months while I looked for a new job. I volunteered
multiple places during this time, to the benefit of these organizations
and to myself. I volunteered at Creekside Elementary School, which
was around the corner from me, and at the Women's Health Center,
close by at UNC–Chapel Hill. While volunteering for Strong Women
Organizing Outrageous Projects (SWOOP), I was helping work on
a home project of painting and landscaping in downtown Durham.

I was talking with another volunteer, who after hearing of my
background and learning I was looking for a job, suggested I try Kel-
ley Services, a contract agency in nearby Research Triangle Park. A
few weeks after applying with them I was placed in a contract position at Duke Center for Health Policy Research. After my contract
was up six months later, the center was pleased with my work and
hired me full-time. I was good at it, as the process was similar to
research I had done before. But the content of the work was very different from what I was accustomed to. The aspects of health policy
were to me dull and tedious. After less than a year of working there, I
began to consider other options.

My supervisor, Pam, had been informed that funding for her
position was ending so she started interviewing elsewhere at Duke.
The world of research and grant funding can mean quick and sudden
career moves that aren't necessarily related to performance. Fortunately for me, it was time for Pam's annual visit with her doctor. Her

doctor was at the campus medical clinic and told her about an open position for a research study focused on diabetes prevention in the Durham community. Pam put me in touch with her since she knew this was up my alley and we both interviewed for the position. Neither of us got it, but she was sure I'd be perfect for another study she was involved with at her clinic on Duke's campus. I interviewed for that one and was hired by the Center for Personalized Medicine at Duke in 2008.

During this time, Julie, one of my best friends, had moved 20 miles east to Raleigh. Our friendship started out in 2001 at the School of Nursing where I worked and she was getting her degree and living on campus in Chapel Hill. Then she just happened to move into an apartment near my house in Durham. Over the next 10 years she moved across Durham, to Winston Salem for graduate school, and then to Virginia in 2009. During this time, we occasionally saw each other and our contact was sporadic at best.

Julie moved back to Chapel Hill in 2012. She had accepted a position at UNC weeks after I had separated from Sean. When she returned, Juliette was two and Alex and Kendall were both four, so we made a fantastic faux family. Eleven years into a solid friendship we had both been there for each other during life-changing moments for both of us, including the deaths of Julie's father, my brother Scott, and her stepson Tomas, who was only 20. We each had been through the wringer enough that we depended on each other more than we ever had before. There was so much more at stake now too, with our kids counting on us to help guide their way.

I was helping her unpack boxes at her townhouse in Southern Village in Chapel Hill, and we were talking about spirituality. Julie picked up *The Four Agreements* by Miguel Ruiz from the bookshelf at the edge of her kitchen where we were talking. She told me the upshot of the book, and she demanded that I take it home and read it. One of the few similarities Julie and I shared was our ideas about spirituality. The book resonated deeply with me as I read it cover to cover. I wholeheartedly believed what I read and honestly applied what I had learned from it in my everyday life. It had become my

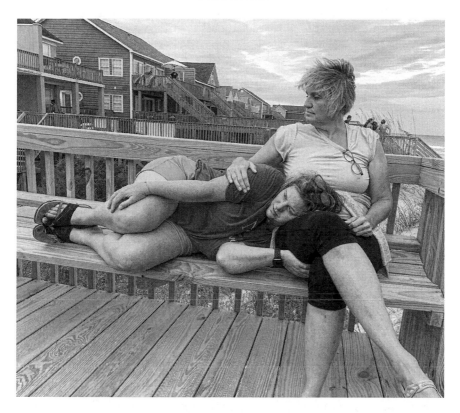

Julie Hughes and Dana Creighton at our annual summer vacation at Topsail Beach in North Carolina, 2019. Julie was sick.

Bible. *The Four Agreements* are (1) be impeccable with your word; (2) don't take anything personally; (3) don't make assumptions; and (4) always do your best. For the next five years I would pick it up and read randomly; it didn't matter what section. It always provided some relevance to whatever situation drew me to it to begin with.

Five years after our divorce, it finally occurred to me that Sean could have *never* been the person that I needed him to be. What I needed was someone that could have fulfilled all my needs, which included helping me figure out and tell my own story. I had learned how to find what I needed by discovering in each of my relationships how I could find even minute gains in my search for answers. One

161

person was not capable of providing all that I needed. Each personal connection that I made over the last 30-plus years gave me a valuable piece of the information that I was searching for. And while I was searching for answers for my own benefit, I tried to affect others' stories in positive ways.

For every crazy, serendipitous moment described, there were at least four or five fall-on-my-face moments that just didn't quite pan out. I also knew from years working in research that learning from our failures can be just as important as our successes. I am vocal and adamant that what I have experienced throughout my life has attributed to my "good fortune." But as strong as I believe this, so is my conviction that the story I tell myself about what may have helped and why, I wholeheartedly believe. After gathering all the pieces, what emerged after looking at everything together told me a more meaningful story than looking at how those same events happened independently.

TRIPLE THREAT

Throughout my life, I had been making connections through my subconscious desires all along, connecting to not only people, but through my career, music, books and even my thoughts and visions that would ultimately allow me to write my story. Connecting with John Evans was integral because his vision that I needed to write down my story was something he saw before I could imagine it. I am quite confident that many of the parenting tools my mom and dad used helped me thrive in less than optimal circumstances. I also realized that, beginning at the age of nine, through the game of basketball, my dad subconsciously began to help shape my brain to defend what my life might have in store for me. It took a couple of years, after finishing graduate school but I eventually caught on.

I was not only the baby in my family but the only girl. I grew up with my dad's strong presence, and I was close with him. Dad was affectionate with me and the love I felt from him never waned. We shared more similarities and interests as I grew up, which only strengthened our bond. He was my first role model and fortunately I would live my life emulating both his spirit and fierce work ethic. My dad had, without using these words or structure, taught me from an early age that I had the ability to

1. create a vision of what I want to achieve;
2. develop a clear path to my goal;
3. make significant sacrifices; and
4. take action to make it happen.

Throughout my life I had gone through each of the four steps in order to get what I wanted—a basketball career, a family, a life with fulfillment, and to love and be loved. My dad's passion for exercise and biology shaped my worldview as I chose exercise physiology as a career. I learned that using research methods to analyze data can help shed light on the variables affecting a condition. My experience as an athlete through college and my education and work experience gave me a better understanding of and insights into how interventions can affect well-being. This quote from Deepak Chopra sums up what my father had been conveying to me and had been reinforced during my research career.

> The mind/body connection is like a telephone line—many telephone lines, in fact, teeming with information. Small things like drinking an orange juice with pulp or eating an apple is being received like a telephone call to your genes. Every thought, everything you eat, every single little thing can tweak your genes activity towards healing.

There is a basketball term I learned at a young age. *Triple threat position* is where you want to be any time you have the ball in your hands. You should be able to put the ball in a position so that you are able at any moment to pass it to someone who is in a better position than you are to dribble or shoot. My triple threat position has evolved over the years, where I put myself in the best position I can.

My life has been a recreation of my mom's life in that every variable that she had working against her are the same variables that allowed me to thrive. Now my triple threat position includes maintaining strong family connections, building meaningful relationships and having a purpose in life.

Only now can I begin to understand and even feel some of the pain and discomfort my mom felt during the last part of her life. I do not feel that doctors she saw had even an ounce of ill will toward my mom. She took the information she was given, and along with her own horrific experience of what this disease had done to her family, Mom created a self-fulfilling prophecy for herself. She would die broken and all alone. But the few things she still had the ability to control would not remain hers much longer, and she knew that. Mom originally felt guilt and then it turned into shame. Guilt is feeling responsible for something happening. Brené Brown, LMSW, Ph.D., states that shame grows exponentially with three things—silence, secrecy and judgment. What can douse this wicked triad is empathy. These are my own thoughts, simulating what may have been playing on repeat in my mom's mind.

> *I'm going to spare them having to watch what is happening to me and spare myself from watching what is starting to happen in Todd and may begin to happen in the others. My life is ruined, and I have ruined my entire family's life. Someone must be at fault for this, and it must be mine. I have no purpose to live anymore.*

I will never know if my simulation is anywhere near what Mom went through. She was so entrenched in her own agony that she would have no way of knowing what was happening across the pond. During the last ten years of her life, Dr. Anita Harding, a British neurologist, was making a dent in the diagnoses of hereditary Ataxias. She was the first person to begin to classify the Ataxias in the 1980s. Unfortunately, this was before the emergence of the Internet. I learned about who Dr. Harding was from the Ataxia Center in Minneapolis just a couple of years ago.

I decided to take a couple of days off work to participate in a research study at the University of Minnesota in Minneapolis. This was in 2012 and I found it posted on the NAF website (Ataxia.org). They have one of the few Ataxia centers, and they were recruiting subjects for a study. The study would provide travel, hotel costs, and a small stipend for participating. It included a motor-skills assessment as well as an MRI. Diane was the research coordinator. She and I really hit it off while I was there for my visit and we kept in touch consistently but sporadically.

Five years later, I was no longer working at Duke and I called Diane. She told me they were doing a follow up, so I scheduled my visit for September of 2017. I also asked her if I could schedule some time to talk to the director of the Ataxia center while I was there. After the clinical visit, I met with Dr. Khalaf Bushara, a neurologist and director of the Bob Allison Ataxia Research Foundation. We talked for only about 30 minutes, and he provided answers to my questions as well as giving me completely new information. He offered that his colleagues Matt Bauer, a genetic counselor, and Dr. Larry Schut, a neurologist, would be thrilled to talk to me about the history of Ataxia research—and they were. Dr. Schut's family was also assaulted by Ataxia although he and his immediate family were spared.

Dr. Schut would see patients at a free clinic in Sioux Falls, South Dakota, to help determine if their symptoms were due to cerebellar degeneration in December 1970. He even treated his own uncle, Dr. John Schut, who helped found the National Ataxia Foundation in 1957 and devoted his life to finding a cure for the same disease that killed him. My mom would have never believed that there were people like Dr. Harding and a pair of Dr. Schuts that, in her lifetime, were out there trying to help people with a family disease like ours. Dr. Larry Schut would also share directly with me how his perspective and experience could inform and add to my story.

Narrative Medicine

Knowing all of this now, after piecing together verbal accounts and looking at medical records along with Mom's own correspondence, I can see how she ended up exactly where she was—sitting in a world where not a single person she had a connection with knew anything about what she was going through. By the time of her diagnosis, unfortunately, the doctors had delivered the last bit of news they had. This is your diagnosis but there is nothing more we can offer you. *You are on your own* is the only thing Mom heard. When you walk into a medical facility asking for something specific, generally they find it or find something to give to you. Mom's experience was that they gave her the information that was spun in a way that *they thought* suited her in that situation.

There are dozens of things I can imagine that Mom could have done differently to help her prevent some of the anguish she went through. I also cannot imagine being in her shoes and then suddenly having the capacity to shift gears and implement a brand-new set of conditions. She was building a family for nearly a decade under the assumption that she would be spared affliction. I can now give her the benefit of the doubt that she was in fact doing her absolute best. And the providers she saw were doing what they felt was warranted. I still have faith that there are lessons to be learned on both sides. In my conversations with others, I believe that being heard can make a huge impact. Telling someone what is important and why can be transformative. Explaining and understanding how we relate to our situation will also begin to shift intentions toward our specific desires.

I wish that Mom could have had the words to express how her purpose on this earth was to be a good mother. In her mind, she had made a series of decisions that put all four of her children at risk for a life-altering condition. I wish her doctors had the permission to ask her what the most important things to her were. All her eggs were in one basket and this container eventually crumbled. In light of a drastically different landscape of today's world, the resources available for many conditions have broadened. Since 1970 when my parents visited the Mayo Clinic both technology and the roles of clinicians have changed drastically.

Over time it became clear that too many responsibilities were being expected from one person. This is exactly why genetic counseling departed from the provider who was delivering clinical information. Doctors giving genetic counseling (GC) advice became separate and independent from clinical care during the 1970s and was not established until the early 1980s. The goal of providing GC was to provide care and recommendations that was *separate from clinical care and not directive.* So now the clinical care remains with the provider and the genetic counseling is provided by someone specially trained in the many issues surrounding specific conditions.

Individuals are invariably going to be blindsided by their own or a family member's changing health or even addiction. I'm no expert on addiction but one obstacle that can complicate its consequences are that the observer and user do not share the same perspective. Family members view and highlight the destructive behaviors observed, but users are only acting on and responding to their pain being soothed. Johann Hari gave a TED Talk in 2015 pointing out that the methods used in the United States to punish addicts actually present barriers to their recovery. By isolating and shaming drug users, we are also overlooking the reasons why they end up there in the first place. Providing connections to a greater purpose and reaching out to the person who relies on genuine love that is bound to the human and not the behavior may help counteract the drive to use. Humans are wired to make and build bonds when we are happy and healthy. In states of disharmony we will bond with anything that substitutes for feelings of unconditional love.

Making healthcare decisions based on our experiences and beliefs rather than "a vs. b" treatment options have a more meaningful impact. It can give the patient ownership in creating a plan that is built on their own frame. Narrative medicine is an approach that is being used to inform others of the unique path down our road. Our experience within the framework of illness is essential to our capacity to endure it. One of the leaders in writing about narrative medicine is Rita Charon of Columbia University. She explains how narratives can strengthen and deepen patient and provider relationships.

> A scientifically competent medicine alone cannot help a patient grapple with the loss of health and find meaning in illness and dying. Along with their growing expertise, doctors need the expertise to listen to their patients, to understand as best they can the ordeals of illness, to honor the meanings of their patients' narratives and be moved by what they behold so that they can act on the patients' behalf [*Narrative Medicine* 3].

This only scratches the surface of what can be accomplished when supplementing providers' expertise with meaningful narratives. In *Narrative Medicine: Honoring the Stories of Illness* Charon identifies and outlines what it is, how to develop narrative competence and the dividends it creates. Not everyone reacts to the same medication or certain types of therapy in the same way. I could not have been more surprised to have gotten any benefits at all from writing about my life, the writing experience I had started with and focused on traumatic events. Being able to tell my story to John has created a dialogue on how we can attain more effective communication. Learning to talk about what is important is a requirement of knowing what is crucial for each of us. Practice talking with someone you trust or consider writing in order to express your true desires.

One of my last duties in research was to be the point of contact to oversee enrollment for patients at Duke and a handful of other health systems across the country for a family history study. A program was designed to take adults' detailed health history and turn it into very specific medical recommendations directed at primary doctors to use in their care. Everyone was different—some uncovered their families health history to assist the program as much as possible, others searched exhaustively to find very little relevant data, and some would have liked to but could not find the time to devote to this task. These participants still got age- and gender-based recommendations that in combination with limited family history information produced guidelines to cast a wider net of conditions to screen for. The providers of the study participants were not obligated to use the recommendations provided.

But it did initiate a conversation where a communal decision could be made to act or not. The tool wasn't a perfect fit for everyone, but it was a starting point to begin thinking about doing things differently than they have always been done. Slowly but surely changes happen and new ways to tackle old barriers emerge. Dozens of participants from across the country called me for some aspect of technical support with this online tool. A high percentage of them also volunteered to share part of their family history with me. It was not part of my job duty to inquire how their family history affected them, but many were compelled to tell me how and why it was important to them.

In my case, all of my providers gave me pieces of the puzzle that have added up to creating a plan that is best for me. Not a single provider gave me the information that made a difference. No doctor referred me to the provider that changed the ground rules. Much to my surprise a health coach was the ringleader who turned my story into a much-needed lesson. I got a new perspective on a life story that wasn't altered by facts but by the meaning attached to it. He had an agenda that was not connected to any medical code that would designate that what he provided met my needs. He listened to what I was saying and responded to my questions with wholehearted discussions related to what was important to me and why.

This can be a template for how providers can gauge if they are giving attention to how their patients experience their journey. Given the time restraints of the medical system it is not a simple request. The fact is that all pertinent conversations likely cannot be addressed by a single provider. There are so many variables that can affect each scenario that may well fall outside the purview of the primary provider. As rapidly as technology advances, the humans involved in providing and receiving the information must also adapt. Otherwise the advantages gained by having a wider bandwidth will fail to reach the intended target. Integration of digital medical records makes access to pertinent information available to multiple providers. This alone will only allow for that information to be available and usable, so the onus still falls on the clinician to deliver care in a way that suits the patient best. Ownership of managing the plan to take from there falls to those providing healthcare.

It was in 2010 when I attended my first NAF meeting in Chicago, after I had been diagnosed in late 2006. Looking back, I can see how the entire group's energy attached to the fragments of my deep desire to help others feeling lost or unheard. This year the 63rd NAF annual conference in Denver was cancelled due to coronavirus. Some of my closest Ataxia-affected friends from Boston and Chicago to Portland reached out to communicate the disappointment of missing this opportunity to connect with members of our tribe. The keynote address was still available to watch on a webinar, but the connections with fellow humans who truly understand each other will have to wait another year.

We are a very fortunate group to have a community of not only individuals but also doctors who dedicate a weekend each year to inform each other of progress in research and ever-changing needs. Last year in Las Vegas a doctor engaged with a roomful of individuals with SCA about how a variety of strategies can be of assistance. This included a discussion about the use of cannabis and CBD oil. Not addressing an issue at all does not change the fact that some people with Ataxia find one or the other useful for a variety of reasons. Providers like this who deeply listen to their patients in order to understand their situation gives me hope that things are moving in the right direction. Talking about the realities of life we each face opens the mind to additional steps we can make to live optimally.

USING OUR WORDS

From an early age, I followed the lead of the rest of my family to remain quiet. This was a piece of cake for me as I was excruciatingly shy anyway. One of the things that John enabled me to overcome was my feeling of being resigned to stay silent. While I spent years hearing silence about this condition, I envisioned living with hope. If you are fortunate enough to not have illness or addiction touch your inner circle almost certainly loss will emerge. Loss is inevitable and is what makes being human so valuable and precious. Trying to avoid or reduce our grieving will only delay feeling the loss. Think of the depth of your pain as it relates to the magnitude of love you had for this person. Loss is sudden but your love is eternal. Carrying on the spirit of the person lost can even strengthen our love, as I have found out.

After I mistakenly thought I was almost done writing, in the fall of 2017 I went to the bookstore to check out memoirs I had meant to read over the last few months. One of them was *It's Not Yet Dark* by Simon Fitzmaurice, a young filmmaker from Ireland who was diagnosed with ALS in 2010 and given four years to live. This was published in 2014, and Simon was still here. In Ireland, patients with ALS typically are not given the option of having home ventilation, but Simon both wanted and needed it and luckily his insurance covered the costs.

> I am not a tragedy. I neither want nor need pity. I am full of hope. The word hope and ALS do not go together in this country. Hope is not about looking for a cure to a disease. Hope is a way of living. We often think we are entitled to a Coca-Cola life. But life is a privilege, not a right. I feel privileged to be alive. That's hope.
>
> It's not important that you know everything about where I come from. About who I am. It is not important you know everything about ALS, about the specifics of the disease, about what it's like to have it. It's only important to remember that behind every disease is a person [91–92].

Reading this, I felt a comradery with him, not because of our similar neurologic pathology, but because of my intense desire to be seen as the person I have always been and not my diagnosis. Through writing I was able to develop a language to talk about this condition and articulate how it affected my family. I also have patterns of thinking that are deeply ingrained and consistently battle against more clear reasoning. Now I am more likely to release my hold on my fears more quickly. My entire life I had learned to muscle through the discomfort that presented itself in numerous ways. Every time that my family was silent about this disease or its effects on us, my internal unrest became more challenging. As an adult my mind was emotionally still a child's, as I continuously thought about but had suppressed talking about the elephant following me from room to room.

My story exemplifies how easily the mind can and will attach itself to building a story that it is fed, then, as time goes by, get bogged down in the minutia of life which can include significant hardships, making it harder to resist listening to this narrative. Personal struggles can too often remain hidden from others and become overwhelming. If we are lucky enough, we can set ourselves up to manage an illness before its symptoms overwhelm us. We can accept and embrace our reality rather than resisting it. Part of my mom's resistance to her reality was born not from misdiagnosis but from different doctors who told her there was nothing wrong. Mom was mortified and frozen by fear when she finally had enough data to discern the risk that we all faced. The doctors Mom saw presented a strong case for her to go on living her life without factoring in the possibility of her eventual diagnosis. With limited evidence to suggest otherwise, they gave mom a Hail Mary pass. She was nowhere near in position to receive it.

The mind operates as the control tower that will handle the flow of rough air by directing it to distant places where it won't cause a major disturbance. This is a coping mechanism but not a very effective one. We shouldn't feel ashamed if we recognize this has been a familiar way to deal with our problems. It usually begins on a subconscious level, so it's no wonder that we feel hijacked. Thought patterns align to make sense of the story regardless of whether the facts are incorrect or missing. We take in and digest new information only as it relates to our perceptions and past experiences. My life was fortunately filled with opportunities that would allow me to be in a far better position than my mom was. When I got called into the game, I devised my own strategy from quietly watching on the sidelines.

I turned 46 this year and I have adapted to declining but manageable symptoms at least for now. However, I recently lost my balance getting up and walking to my bedroom door to let my dog out. It was nearly midnight, so I had been asleep for two hours. When I pivoted on the wood floor after opening the door, my momentum was driving me forward but my feet lost track of where the ground was. The combination of the darkness of night and my sudden change in direction resulted in my entire sense of balance being held hostage. No light in the room left one entire sense almost useless, and the remaining ones, which would typically step up and take over, were only partially alert and collectively not enough to stay upright.

I crashed hard, but I got up with only a goose egg on the back of my head and a bruised ego. The next day I told Kendall that the unsteadiness of my walking was increased by the darkness. That is why I fell, and this is the way I keep her informed of this illness. Explaining to her what she sees, hears or feels that warrants a practical explanation to how she may or may not be affected. In this case, it does not affect her that I lost my balance and fell except that my loud crash landing woke her up. It does affect Kendall that she knows that I am including her in a continuous dialogue. She suggested that I get a nightlight in my room.

I have made this and other accommodations to live my life in a way that suits me. I recently went to a medical device retailer and test-drove a gait trainer. Think of how a walker is used but in reverse. This will provide support on walks like at nearby Duke Forest when I want to conserve my energy and avoid getting physically drained while navigating uneven terrain or at a conference when extended periods of start and stop walking can be especially exhausting. My energy and stamina as well as my abilities are continually diminishing. I will also utilize stability poles and grab bars in my house before it is required. When in public I carry a single trekking pole as a signal to others that I need more space or time. People will more often than not hold the door for me. It also provides another sensory input to my brain that remains in contact with the ground as I walk. I grab hold of someone's arm no matter if it's a good friend or just an acquaintance, borrowing a piece of their stability. Connecting to others surrounding me is a tool I have found invaluable, physically and emotionally, and this usually does not even require any words be exchanged.

Using our words seems so basic yet it cannot be accomplished if we don't practice and even fumble through trying. I think all parents can remember when their children were small and still learning how to communicate. We naturally give young children the benefit of the doubt, knowing they will need numerous attempts to articulate what they need. There are still many medical professionals who are not familiar with a particular condition or what effects it can have on families. *Surely no one else could begin to understand, so why even try to reach out for any help?* There are stories we each have to tell that give others the chance to hear what is important to each of us. Isn't that what should guide the decisions of how to proceed next?

Whether it be a discussion about family planning or about what end of life choice is right, if we can provide a context to what the most important things to us are, that can provide a foundation for a more complex and in-depth discussion that should preface life-altering conversations and decisions. Talking about and then confronting hard conversations surrounding illness, mortality and loss can benefit both sides. Completely understanding someone else is not required but fully hearing and listening can begin to help someone find their words. These words can in turn lead to better understanding for everyone. Try to stay focused on talking about what you hold dear. Every important conversation should start from there.

Appendix A: Correspondence Regarding the Family Disease

Correspondence on next five pages.

Appendix A

204 S. Tyner Drive
Warsaw, Indiana 46580
December 30, 1970

Genetic Counseling Service
Mayo Clinic
Rochester, Minn. 55901

Gentlemen:

I would like some information concerning whether or not genetic counseling service can be obtained by correspondence or if a visit to the clinic is necessary? Perhaps more information could help you determine this.

Several members of my wife's family have gradually become victims of Friedreich's ataxia (her father, three brothers and one sister).

My wife and I have two sons (ages 8 and 6) who were born just prior to the time when the ataxia in my wife's family was first being diagnosed. We planned no more children, mainly because of the hereditary question of which we knew very little.

However, my wife is now eight weeks pregnant and we are very concerned about the hereditary condition of the unborn. Can it be predicted what chance there will be of my wife and our two sons being affected and now our unborn. Can anything be done in any of the circumstances.

We can supply further information including reports from my wife's father's doctor, autopsy report on the deceased brother and other information. You may call us collect at Warsaw, Indiana, (219) 267-6551.

Sincerely,

Robert Creighton

Correspondence Regarding the Family Disease

Marge's letter to her nieces and nephews

January 25, 1983

Dear Vickie,
Dear Rick,

Grandma sent me Pam's letter in which she asked for addresses and more information. I realized that you(nieces and nephews), although you know a lot about the disease symptoms by personal observation, probably know little about some of the things that really concern you. I have asked lots of questions and will share with you what I know. I must warn you though that the doctors can't give definite answers because they don't know. They are very evasive. When you write for information, what do you call the disease? Prior to 1971, we thought it was Friedrich's Ataxia. When I went to Mayo's in 1971, they said it had no name but could be called the Poynter Disease because each family has symptoms that are unique. On a paper from I.U. on Carolyn in 1974, they have written Friedrick's Ataxia? In 1980, when I went to Bluffton, Indiana, Clinic the doctor called it Olivo-Ponto-Cerebellar Atrophy Type IV.

It appears that I will probably have a milder case since I'm having it later than others in my generation. So, don't panic if you think you are having some symptoms. I think the same would probably apply to you. You wouldn't have as strong a case as Mike and Susan. Besides, the disease does not start with wheelchairs. At 30 I had some symptoms which I was sure confirmed that I had it. They said I didn't. At 40 I had some more symptoms. They still said no. Now at 42, they think the symptoms are the disease. Twelve years ago, I was sure I had it (and I did) and I'm still walking around.

The worst thing for me is knowing that I've already passed it on to 1, 2, or 3 of my 4 children and the severity of the disease for them is an open question. If I felt they could be 40 before they were seriously affected it wouldn't be so bad. Maybe the heredity question has never been explained to you. If a parent has it each child has a 50-50 chance of developing it. That's just like flipping a coin. All the children could have it. None could have it. But it's more likely to be some of each. If you as parents turn out to have it, your children also carry the possibility. If you do not have it, your kids do not have to worry. The trouble is deciding whether or not you have it. Conceivably, you could be 40 or 50, and by then your own children may have already passed it on to children. But that would be the exception. The thing the doctors kept telling me was that I would be expected to have a case similar to others in my generation. I would recommend that you think strongly before having any more children of your own and possibly passing it on. You are much safer than my children because of your age. My kids are going to have to consider carefully having children at all.

Earl's father had it. Also, Grandpa had one brother who also had it. This brother had one daughter who did not have it, so it ended there. Earl had two brother who did not have it. So it ended there. It's only in Earl's family except for a first cousin of Earls' in Brownsburg, Ind. who has it. So apparently, there is some misinformation way back.

I hope I have provided some information. I will probably be seeing the doctors again so if you have more questions which I can't answer I could ask for you. I need to know specifically what your questions are.

Again, don't panic. There are sometimes that I have difficulty believing that anything is wrong with me. Write if you have more questions.

Marge

CN

CAYLOR-NICKEL RESEARCH FOUNDATION, Inc.

Telephone A/C 219 824-3500 • • • Bluffton, Indiana 46714

September 11, 1980

Sam Rhine, MD
2400 N Tibbs Ave
Indianapolis, IN 46222

Dear Dr Rhine:

Mrs Robert Creighton was seen for counseling on September 5, 1980. The patient was most concerned over the inheritance of and clinical findings associated with olivopontocerebellar atrophy IV. Affected family members include the patient's grandfather, father, and 4 siblings, all of whom are deceased. Disease onset occurred in the father at age 40 years; the sibs developed symptoms in their 20's.

As Mrs Creighton approached age 40 without symptoms, she reports feeling relieved at having escaped the disease. Recently, however, she has become alarmed over isolated instances of staggering and poor coordination. The patient was quite alarmed over the implications for herself as well as her 4 children.

A physical examination was performed by Dr Patricia Bader, and a neurological examination by Dr. John Bossard. Both of these evaluations were well within normal limits. It is our opinion that Mrs Creighton is not exhibiting the initial stages of a degenerative disease. Considerable time was spent discussing these findings with the patient and reassuring her. We feel that the visit served to relieve much of Mrs Creighton's anxiety.

Sincerely,

Patricia I Bader, MD
Director of Clinical Research

PIB:nc
cc: Medical Records
    Mrs Creighton

Fort Wayne
Medical Laboratory
Corporation

LKY-6636
Loh.

500 Medical Center Bldg
Fort Wayne, Indiana 46801-026(
Phone (219) 423-152(

K. R. SCHLADEMAN, M.D.
Director Emeritus

J. A. FOSTER, M.D.
Director of Laboratories,
Fort Wayne Medical Laboratory

C. M. FRANKHOUSER, M.D.
Director of Laboratories,
Parkview Memorial Hospital

**BLOOD BANKING
and COAGULATION**
R. Gangadhar, M.D.

CLINICAL CHEMISTRY
D. Smith, M.D.

**CLINICAL GENETICS
and CYTOGENETICS**
P. I. Bader, M.D.

**ELECTRON MICROSCOPY
and CYTOLOGY**
S. Sage Lee, M.D., Ph.D.

FORENSIC PATHOLOGY
C. M. Frankhouser, M.D.

HEMATOLOGY
J. A. Foster, M.D.

SURGICAL PATHOLOGY
R. Burkhardt, M.D.

CONSULTING STAFF

ENDOCRINOLOGY
Soja Park Bennett, M.D.

MICROBIOLOGY
Benjamin Becker, Ph.D.

BUSINESS MANAGER
Donald Evers

COORDINATORS

MARKETING & PERSONNEL
Mario J. Palmer

TECHNICAL EQUIPMENT
Andrew Weber

CONTRACTED SERVICES
Thomas Bubb

LABORATORY SERVICES
David Hablitzel, M.T.

Mrs. Marjorie Creighton was first seen by me on September 5, 1980. A: that time she was concerned over the possible inheritance of Olivo-ponto-cerebellar atrophy type IV. Several of her family member: have been affected, including her grandfather, her father, four siblir and each of these individuals is now deceased. In addition, Mrs. Creighton states that at least four of her nieces and nephews wei affected by this problem.

The disease onset usually begins in the third decade and the disease usually progesses over 5 - 10 years before death. Her father, howevei developed his disease in his 40's and died in his 60's. When I first saw Mrs. Creighton in 1980, she discussed some episodes of staggering and poor coordination. She was quite alarmed because of the implications for herself as well as her four children. I examined Mrs. Creighton and was concerned at that time that her voice was somewhat harsh, that she showed some difficulty in walking a straight line and hopping. I asked her to see Dr. John Bossard who felt that h exam was within normal limits. Consequently, I told Mrs. Creighton th I felt she was not exhibiting the initial stages of a degenerative disease. Mrs. Creighton returned home and during the next two years noticed some progression of her difficulties. She had problems on rising from the sitting position, she had trouble with balance, she noticed that when she was walking she would begin to fall sideways, she noticed difficulty in going up and down stairs, especially without a banister. She realized her trouble with balance was when she was lacking confidence. However, she felt that the problem was getting worse within the last two years.

On physical exam in 1982, again, I noticed some left-sided weakness, some dyspraxia of speech, some problems with the finger-to-nose test, a reasonably good ability in the heel-to-shin test. Her Romberg was normal. There was no problem with sensory or vibration. She, again, however, showed very poor ability to walk a straight line and she coulc not hop at all.

On Mrs. Creighton's first visit I felt that many of her difficulties might have had an emotional overlay, simply because she had just reache age 40 which was the age her father was diagnosed at. However, on second exam, I felt it would be worthwhile to have Mrs. Creighton examined by an neurologist. I did refer her to Dr. Stanley Wissman. I understand that Dr. Wissman feels she has a positive neurological examination. She is to return in two weeks for further evaluation and will also come by my office to discuss the implications in terms of inheritance and in terms of her family's particular prospects.

Patricia I. Bader, M.D., Director
Northeast Indiana Genetic
Counseling Center
Parkview Memorial Hospital
Fort Wayne, IN 46805

PIB:sm

"A **QUALITY** laboratory since **1905**"

Appendix A

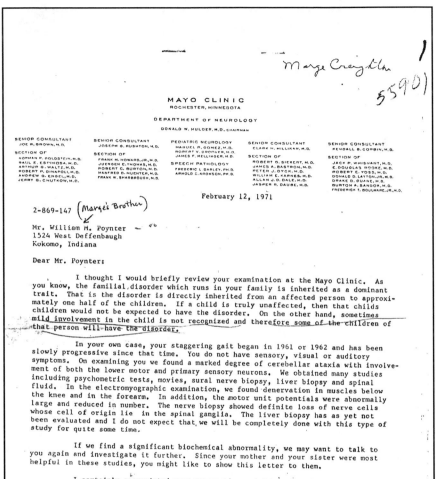

Marge Creighton
5590)

MAYO CLINIC
ROCHESTER, MINNESOTA

DEPARTMENT OF NEUROLOGY
DONALD W. MULDER, M.D., CHAIRMAN

SENIOR CONSULTANT	SENIOR CONSULTANT	PEDIATRIC NEUROLOGY	SENIOR CONSULTANT	SENIOR CONSULTANT
JOE R. BROWN, M.D.	JOSEPH G. RUSHTON, M.D.	MANUEL R. GOMEZ, M.D.	CLARK H. MILLIKAN, M.D.	KENDALL B. CORBIN, M.D.
		ROBERT V. GROOVER, M.D.		
SECTION OF	SECTION OF	JAMES F. MELLINGER, M.D.	SECTION OF	SECTION OF
NORMAN P. GOLDSTEIN, M.D.	FRANK M. HOWARD, JR., M.D.		ROBERT G. SIEKERT, M.D.	JACK P. WHISNANT, M.D.
RAUL E. ESPINOSA, M.D.	JUERGEN C. THOMAS, M.D.	SPEECH PATHOLOGY	JAMES A. BASTRON, M.D.	E. DOUGLAS ROOKE, M.D.
ARTHUR G. WALTZ, M.D.	ROBERT C. BURTON, M.D.	FREDERIC L. DARLEY, PH.D.	PETER J. DYCK, M.D.	ROBERT E. YOSS, M.D.
ROBERT P. DINAPOLI, M.D.	MANFRED D. MUENTER, M.D.	ARNOLD C. ARONSON, PH.D.	WILLIAM E. KARNES, M.D.	DONALD D. LAYTON, JR., M.D.
ANDREW G. ENGEL, M.D.	FRANK W. SHARBROUGH, M.D.		ALLAN J. D. DALE, M.D.	DRAKE D. DUANE, M.D.
JERRY G. CHUTKOW, M.D.			JASPER R. DAUBE, M.D.	BURTON A. SANDOK, M.D.
				FREDERICK T. BOULWARE, JR., M.D.

February 12, 1971

2-869-147 *(Marge's Brother)*

Mr. William M. Poynter — *46*
1524 West Deffenbaugh
Kokomo, Indiana

Dear Mr. Poynter:

I thought I would briefly review your examination at the Mayo Clinic. As you know, the familial disorder which runs in your family is inherited as a dominant trait. That is the disorder is directly inherited from an affected person to approximately one half of the children. If a child is truly unaffected, then that childs children would not be expected to have the disorder. On the other hand, sometimes mild involvement in the child is not recognized and therefore some of the children of that person will have the disorder.

In your own case, your staggering gait began in 1961 or 1962 and has been slowly progressive since that time. You do not have sensory, visual or auditory symptoms. On examining you we found a marked degree of cerebellar ataxia with involvement of both the lower motor and primary sensory neurons. We obtained many studies including psychometric tests, movies, sural nerve biopsy, liver biopsy and spinal fluid. In the electromyographic examination, we found denervation in muscles below the knee and in the forearm. In addition, the motor unit potentials were abnormally large and reduced in number. The nerve biopsy showed definite loss of nerve cells whose cell of origin lie in the spinal ganglia. The liver biopsy has as yet not been evaluated and I do not expect that we will be completely done with this type of study for quite some time.

If we find a significant biochemical abnormality, we may want to talk to you again and investigate it further. Since your mother and your sister were most helpful in these studies, you might like to show this letter to them.

I certainly appreciated your cooperation and I hope you found your stay here not too unpleasant.

Best regards.

Sincerely yours,

Peter James Dyck, M.D.

PJD:cb
P.S.: I forgot to mention thatthe final diagnosis that we came to was that of dominantly inherited cerebellar ataxia with involvement of the lower motor and primary sensory neurons.
220 FIRST STREET SOUTHWEST, ROCHESTER, MINNESOTA 55901 • TELEPHONE (507) 282-2511

Appendix B:
Documents Requested and Received from Indiana University School of Medicine– Indianapolis in 1999

Documents on next nine pages.

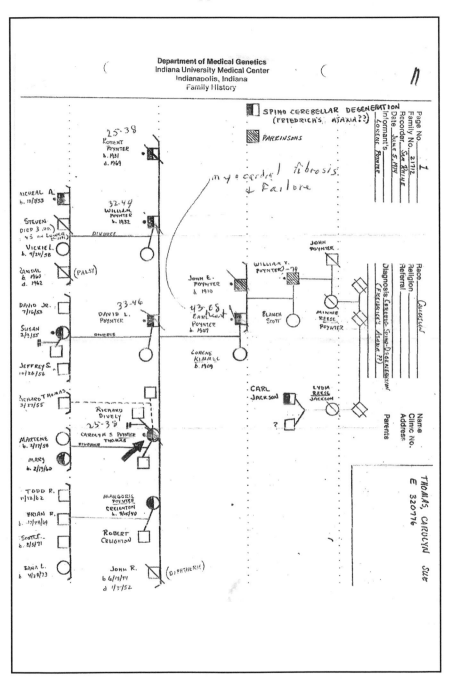

Mayo Clinic

Rochester, Minnesota 55905   Telephone 507 284-2511

Peter James Dyck, M.D.
Department of Neurology

May 17, 1983

2-869-143

Dr. David Haines
Kosiusko Community Hospital
Warsaw, Indiana 46580

Dear Dr. Haines:

Thank you for referring Mrs. Robert Creighton. As you know Mrs. Creighton had been previously seen at Mayo Clinic regarding the possibilities of inherited cerebellar ataxia. At that time there was no evidence by examination of such a disorder, but she of course was at risk.

Her present symptoms consist of loss of balance, which has been slowly progressive for 2½ years. She has difficulty with legibility of her hand writing also for 2 years. Her speech is garbled and indistinct possibly for about 2 years. She complains about running into things, difficulty in climbing up or down stairs, and difficulty with balance in walking and turning around.

Her present height is 5'6"; her weight 145 pounds. She is not taking medications. Her general health is good. She has felt depressed and very worried about her children, lest they get the same disorder that runs in the family.

A detailed kinship history was taken which provides evidence that the disorder is an autosomal dominant with good penetrance. There is considerable variability of the age at onset, and in the rate of worsening.

Dr. Younge saw her in the Eye Department. The vision was good, but she does have some abnormality of eye movement with subtle dysmetria. Dr. Darley saw her in the Speech Department and observed ataxic dysarthria. The muscle strength is generally good. She has ataxia of limb movements, which may be a combination of cerebellar and sensory ataxia. I thought there was also some truncal ataxia. The toes are down-going and she has mechanoreceptor loss in the upper and lower limbs.

183

2-869-143

Dr. David Haines
May 17, 1983
Page 2

   I'm enclosing a copy of the nerve conduction and EMG
sheet which shows relatively good motor nerve conduction
velocities, decreased amplitudes of sensory potentials, and
no evidence of lower motor neuron involvement. I'm also
enclosing a copy of the computer assisted sensory examination
which provides evidence of abnormality for all three types of
sensation on the foot. A monoclonal protein was not detected.
The hexosaminidase A was normal. X-rays of the chest showed
fluid or thickened pleura in the left costophrenic angle. The
sedimentation rate was 15 mm. The hematology group values
were somewhat abnormal being reduced for hemoglobin, erythro-
cyte count, hematocrit count and MCV. The hemoglobin was
10.2 gm/dl. An occult blood was obtained and this was negative.
The chemistry group values were normal. The cholesterol was
at the 5% level. The lipoprotein pattern is normal. Serum
and lymphocytes were taken for glutamate dehydrogenase estima-
tions and if these show abnormality I will let you know. These
will not be run for several months.

   In summary, it is now apparent that Mrs. Creighton does
have a dominantly inherited spinocerebellar degeneration.
Clearly this is not Friedreich's Ataxia because it is dominantly
inherited, and it is not pure olivo-ponto-cerebellar degeneration
because there is evidence of involvement of the peripheral
sensory system. I know that it must be very distressing for Mrs.
Creighton that she was seen here 11 years ago and the diagnosis
was not made at that time. My assumption is that the symptomatic
involvement has developed since that examination. Unfortunately
the markers such as the electromyogram are not sensitive enough
to detect this disorder prior to its symptomatic development.
I do not think there is a specific treatment for this neurologic
disease, but hopefully such will become available soon. The fact
that she has late onset is clearly in her favor. I have discussed a program of physical fitness with her, emphasizing the
need to keep her weight down. I have also encouraged her to
continue going out and carrying on with the important functions
she has as a mother and wife. I believe that she tends to blame
herself unnecessarily, particularly as it relates to her having
children who are at risk for the disorder.

   I enjoyed seeing Mrs. Creighton again. I'm sorry that she
has a difficult disease, but it is one that she can live with and

(rest of letter is
missing ?? - - -)
from file 7/95

MAYO CLINIC
ROCHESTER, MINNESOTA
55901

SECTION OF MEDICAL STATISTICS
EPIDEMIOLOGY AND POPULATION GENETICS
LEONARD T. KURLAND, M.D.
WILLIAM F. TAYLOR, PH.D.
LILA ELVEBACK, PH.D.
HYMIE GORDON, M.D.
FRED T. NOBREGA, M.D.

January 7, 1971

Mr. Robert Creighton
204 E. Tyner Drive
Warsaw, Indiana   46580

Dear Mr. Creighton:

Thank you for your letter of December 30, in which you inquire about
genetics counselling and Friedreich's ataxia.

I am afraid that I cannot help you by letter. Genetics counselling
requires, first of all, precision of diagnosis and I have some doubt
about the diagnosis of Friedreich's ataxia in your wife's family. Usually,
in Friedreich's ataxia, the unsteadiness is well-established by the early
20's; in your wife's family the disease seems to have had a much later
onset.

Apart from the question of diagnosis, genetics counselling usually
requires a great deal of information which is difficult to collect by
mail. It also calls for intimate discussions between the doctor and the
patient, as in any other medical consultation. Accordingly, it would
be much better if you and your wife would come to see me at the Mayo
Clinic. It would be best if one of your wife's affected relatives
(a brother or her father) could attend at the same time so that we can
satisfy ourselves about the diagnosis. Some of my colleagues in Neurology are particularly expert in the ataxic group of diseases and would
provide us with valuable diagnostic opinions. This would add precision
to any genetic counselling that I could give you.

Please let me know if you would like me to make any arrangements for you.

Yours sincerely,

Hymie Gordon, M.D.

HG/sll

lttr includio copy N Unve Blud 550 N. Unve Blud name d bith Rm. 3280 Indy, Ind 46202

274-2286 Health Info Med. Records

FAX
TRANSMISSION

Indiana University School of Medicine
Department of Medical and Molecular Genetics
Medical Research and Library Building Room IB-130
Indiana University Medical Center
975 West Walnut Street
Indianapolis, IN 46202-5251
(317) 274-2241 FAX: (317) 274-2387

DATE: 5/14/99

TO: Dane Creighton

COMPANY:

FAX #: 419 537 5605 TELEPHONE #:

FROM: Phyllis Humphrey — Sarver

FAX #: 317 274-2387 TELEPHONE #: 274-1058

NOTES:

Number of Pages (Including Cover Page): 3

```
FATHER:  Earl S. Poynter  8/19/07-8/25/75  (68)  (Symptoms early 40's)

    1. SON: Robert E. Poynter 2/10/31-5/21/69  (38)  (Symptoms mid 20's)

    2. SON: William M. Poynter 6/4/32-4/28/77  (44)  (    "     mid 20's)

        A. SON: Michael A. Poynter 10/3/53-4/22/84 (30) (Symp. age 12)
        B. SON: Steven Poynter ..................... (3 months )
        C. DAUGHTER: Vickie L. (Poynter) Edwards 4/24/58
           1c. DAUGHTER: Kassie L. Edwards 4/7/76
           2c. SON: James N. Edwards 10/18/77
        D. SON: Randall Poynter ..................... (2 years)

    3. SON: David L. Poynter, Sr. 2/11/34-7/31/80 (46) (Symp. early 30's)

        A. SON: David L. Poynter, Jr. 7/16/53-11/10/80 (27) (accident)
           1a. DAUGHTER: Kara N. Poynter 8/3/73
        B. DAUGHTER: Susan L. (Poynter) Turnpaugh 2/9/55 (Symp. mid teens)
        C. SON: Jeffrey S. Poynter 10/26/56

    4. DAUGHTER: Carolyn S. (Poynter) Thomas 9/29/35-6/22/74 (38) ("  ")

        A. SON: Richard E. Thomas 3/27/55
           1a. DAUGHTER: Melissa T. Thomas 8/21/76
        B. DAUGHTER: Martene R. (Thomas) Bolinger 2/17/58
           1b. DAUGHTER: Hannah L. Bolinger 5/25/85
        C. DAUGHTER: Mary E. Thomas 2/19/60  (Symptoms mid teens)

    5. DAUGHTER: Marjorie A. (Poynter) Creighton 9/15/40 (Symp. late 30's)
        A. SON: Todd R. Creighton 11/12/62
        B. SON: Brian R. Creighton 12/28/64
        C. SON: Eric S. Creighton 8/5/71
        D. DAUGHTER: Dana L. Creighton 4/28/73

    6. SON: John R. Poynter 6/15/44-1/31/52  (7)  (Diptheria)


NOTE: UNCLES OF EARL POYNTER 1.** William V. Poynter (75)  (Parkinsons)
                             2.** Ray Poynter
                             3.** Ralph Poynter              ****

              A.**Daughter: Enid Poynter has symptoms ****
```

Appendix B

Indiana University Hospitals
1100 West Michigan Street
Indianapolis, Indiana 46202

| i/90 | AUTHORIZATION TO OBTAIN MEDICAL INFORMATION | MS188700 | |

SEE REVERSE SIDE FOR INSTRUCTIONS

For the purpose of patient care, I hereby request and authorize:

_____

_____

_____

☐ In-Patient ☐ Out-Patient

to furnish: Department of Medical & Molecular Genetics
Indiana University Medical Center
975 West Walnut Street, IB-130
Indianapolis, Indiana 46202-5251

any medical record information in your medical record files concerning

EARL POYNTER (; other family members) in regards to treatment for olivopontocerebellar
(full name of patient)   degeneration II

— ALL —

(Dates or specific information)

It is understood that this consent is subject to revocation by me (us) at any time except to the extent that action has been taken in reliance thereon. It is also understood that this consent expires 60 days from the

date signed unless otherwise specified _____

Hospital Number _____ Date of Birth _____

Sex ____ Race ____ Maiden Name _____ Mother's Name _____

✶ Address Dana Creighton
2472 Glenwood Ave. Toledo, OH 43620

Date 5/17/99   Signed Dana Creighton

Witness _____ Signed _____
(If above is a minor)

INDIANA UNIVERSITY HOSPITALS' USE ONLY:

When information is received, please notify:

Requesting Physician _____

location _____ extension _____

AUTHORIZATION TO OBTAIN MEDICAL INFORMATION   Y-36

188

TOP IMPRINT MARGIN

FORM TEMP.	INDIANA UNIVERSITY MEDICAL CENTER	

MEDICAL GENETICS

Thomas, Carolyn Sue

Hospital No. E320776

Family No. 21712

June 12, 1974

This 39 year old white woman was admitted to University Hospital for treatment of a chronic progressive neurologic disorder which has been diagnosed as Friedreich's Ataxia There has been multiple affected individuals in the family in a pattern that is consistent with autosomal dominant inheritance. The patient is now severely incapacitated with her disease and is emaciated, bedridden, incontinent and has multiple bed sores. Abnormal movements are a striking feature of the neurologic findings. The patient has rapid protruding movements of the tongue as well as rhythmic flailing movements of the arms and hands. It is easy to see how other family members have been diagnosed as having "Parkinson's Disease" if their findings were similar to those of the patient.

Impression: Dominantly inherited progressive neurologic degenerative disease.

Comment: There are several inherited neurologic disorders associated with abnormalitie of movement which have been characterized at the biochemical level, however most of these conditions such as Wilson's Disease, a-beta-lipoproteinemia, ataxia-telangiectasi and xeroderma pigmentosa, are transmitted as autosomal recessive traits. However it might be worthwhile obtaining ceruloplasmin assays, serum cholesterol, and IgA determinations to document that these findings are normal in the present patient. It might also be worthwhile to obtain electrocardiogram to see whether there are any findings suggestive of Friedreich's cardiomyopathy. I would also recommend a careful opthalmologic examination to search for evidence of retinitis pigmentosa. Several families have been reported in the literature in which a condition resembling Parkinson's Disease has been transmitted as an autosomal dominant trait[1,2,3]. If familial Parkinsonism can be documented in the present family it might be of great interest to search for evidence of altered manganese metabolism in this patient. At least one genetic disorder involving manganese metabolsim has been documented in the laboratory mouse where vestibular dysfunction is a major feature.

Walter E. Nance, M.D., Ph.D.
Professor of Medical Genetics

WEN:ldm

References: 1. Allan, W.: Archives of Internal Medicine 60:424, 1937.
2. Bell, J. and Clark, H.A.: Annals of Eugenics 1:455, 1926.
3. Spellman, G.G.: Journal of American Medical Association 179:372, 1962.

cc: Medical Records

USE ONE SIDE ONLY

MEDICAL GENETICS | 3

FATHER: Earl S. Poynter   8/19/07 - 8/25/75   (68) (Symptoms early 40's)

    SON: Robert E. Poynter 2/10/31 - 5/21/69 (38) " mid 20's) (age 38)

    SON: William M. Poynter 6/4/32 - 4/28/77 (440 " " 20's) (" 44)

       SON: Michael A. Poynter 10/3/53   " age 12

       DAUGHTER: Vickie L.(Poynter) Edwards 4/24/58

           DAUGHTER: Kassie L. Edwards 4/7/76

           SON: James N. Edwards 10/18/77

    SON: David L. Poynter, Sr. 2/11/34 - 7/31/80 (Symptoms early 30's) (age 46)

       SON: David L. Poynter, Jr. 7/16/53 - 11/10/80 (Killed accident) →(" 27)

       Daughter: Kara N. Poynter 8/3/73

       DAUGHTER: Susan L.(Poynter) Turnpaugh 2/9/55 (Symptoms mid teens)

       SON: Jeffrey S. Poynter 10/26/56

  DAUGHTER: Carolyn S.(Poynter) Thomas 9/29/35 - 6/22/74   (age 38)
                            (Symptoms mid teens)

       SON: Richard E. Thomas 3/27/55

        Daughter: Melissa T. Thomas 8/21/76

       DAUGHTER: Martene R. Thomas 2/17/58

       DAUGHTER: Mary E. Thomas (Betsy) 2/19/60   (Symptoms mid teens)

  DAUGHTER: Marjorie A. (Poynter) Creighton 9/15/40 (Symptoms late 30's)

       SON: Todd R. Creighton 11/12/62

       SON: Brian R. Creighton 12/28/64

       SON: Eric S. Creighton   8/5/71

       DAU: Dana L. Creighton 4/28/73

  SON: John R. Poynter 6/15/44 - 1/31/52 (died of Diptheria)

(Marge's Records — Symptoms are guessed)

Bibliography

Books

Brooks, Melanie. *Writing Hard Stories: Celebrated Memoirists Who Shaped Art from Trauma*. Beacon Press, 2017.

Brown, Brené. *Daring Greatly: How the Courage to Be Vulnerable Transforms the Way We Live, Love, Parent, and Lead*. Avery, 2015.

Charon, Rita. *Narrative Medicine: Honoring the Stories of Illness*. Oxford University Press, 2008.

Doidge, Norman. *The Brain That Changes Itself: Stories of Personal Triumph from the Frontiers of Brain Science*. ReadHowYouWant, 2017.

Fitzmaurice, Simon. *It's Not Yet Dark*. Mariner Books/Houghton Mifflin Harcourt, 2018.

Gawande, Atul. *Being Mortal: Illness, Medicine and What Matters in the End*. Profile Books, 2015.

Kapsambelis, Niki. *The Inheritance: A Family on the Front Lines of the Battle Against Alzheimer's Disease*. Simon & Schuster, 2018.

Lesser, Elizabeth. *Broken Open: How Difficult Times Can Help Us Grow*. Ebury Digital, 2010.

Murphy, Joseph. *The Power of Your Subconscious Mind: The Complete Original Edition, Plus Bonus Material*. St. Martin's Essentials, 2019.

Ruiz, Don Miguel. *The Four Agreements*. Hay House, 2008.

Strayed, Cheryl. *Wild: From Lost to Found on the Pacific Crest Trail*. Alfred A. Knopf, 2019.

Wolynn, Mark. *It Didn't Start with You: How Inherited Family Trauma Shapes Who We Are and How to End the Cycle*. Penguin Books, 2017.

Journal Articles

Friedreich, N. "Über Ataxie mit besonderer Berücksichtigung der hereditären Formen" [About ataxia with special reference to hereditary forms]. *Arch Pathol Anat Phys Klin Med* 68, 145–245 (1876). doi:10.1007/BF01879049.

Friedreich, N. "Über degenerative Atrophie der spinalen Hinterstränge" [About degenerative atrophy of the spinal posterior column]. Arch Pathol Anat Phys Klin Med 26, 391–419 (1863). doi:10.1007/BF01930976.

Muth, Christopher C. "ASO Therapy: Hope for Genetic Neurological Diseases." *JAMA* 319, no. 7 (2018). doi:10.1001/jama.2017.18665.

Pulst, Stefan M. "Degenerative Ataxias, from Genes to Therapies." *Neurology* 86, no. 24 (2016). doi:10.1212/wnl.0000000000002777.

Bibliography

Websites

The Ataxian Movie, Life Is About How We React. theataxianmovie.com/.

Brown, Brené. "Shame versus Guilt." https://www.bing.com/videos/search?q=brene+brown+and+shame+silence+and&docid=608003326761700453&mid=48654DCB9BA30049E7C548654DCB9BA30049E7C5&view=detail&FORM=VIRE

Evans, John F., Ed.D. "Write Yourself Well." *Psychology Today*, blog. https://www.psychologytoday.com/us/blog/write-yourself-well.

Hari, Johann. "Everything you think you know about addiction is wrong." Ted Talk.

Heywood, Jamie. Ted Talk. ted.com/talks/jamie_heywood_the_big_idea_my_brother_inspired.

Kalaichandran, Amitha. "Resolving to Be Coached." *New York Times*, 7 Jan. 2020. www.nytimes.com/2020/01/07/well/live/new-years-resolutions-health-fitness-coaching.html

National Ataxia Foundation, Connecting Ataxia families, researchers, clinicians and the community.www.ataxia.org

S.158, A bill to provide that human life shall be deemed to exist from conception. Report, Subcommittee on Separation of Powers to Senate Judiciary Committee S-158, 97th Congress, 1st Session 1981. https://www.congress.gov/bill/97th-congress/senate-bill/158.

So Much, So Fast. Documentary of life of Stephen Heywood.

Ted Radio Hour. Maslow's Hierarchy of Needs. npr.org/programs/ted-radio-hour/399796647/maslows-human-needs.

Index

Index